HEALTHY HORSE
HANDBOOK

HEALTHY HORSE HANDBOOK
The Owner's Illustrated Guide

Fritz Sevelius · Harry Pettersson · Lennart Olsson

Translated by Richard Fleming

David McKay Company, Inc.
New York

CONTENTS

LIST OF ILLUSTRATIONS

PREFACE

Sweden has the reputation of being a country where animals are well treated, and has a long tradition of horsemanship that has survived to the present time, very largely due to the activities of the Swedish army during the period when it was very dependent upon horses.

The old horsemen have almost all gone now, but the tradition is being kept alive by means of courses and demonstrations at the national stud at Flyinge; by a flourishing programme of courses on riding and looking after horses organised by the Swedish Horse Society at Strömsholm; and by the retention of the horse-judging scheme under the auspices of the Department of Agriculture.

The Swedish Warm-blood Horse Society has played an important part in the preservation of the Swedish tradition of horsemanship, notably by its efforts to save the Swedish warm-blood horse, inspired by the legendary Dr Arvid Aaby-Ericsson. Meanwhile it is no doubt an interesting sign of the times that the old horsemen have largely been replaced by horsewomen!

Sweden also has a high international reputation for treatment of disease in horses. The basis for this reputation was the work of John Vennerholm, professor of surgery at the Veterinary Institute in Stockholm at the end of last century. His work was continued by his successor, Gerhard Forssell, who developed techniques of examination and treatment in the early years of this century that did not become general in other parts of the world until 30–40 years later. Eric Åkerblom,

the leading Swedish research worker into diseases of the foot, particularly laminitis, has also played an important part in the development of modern Swedish veterinary treatment of horses.

A lot of other young Swedish veterinary research workers at the Veterinary Institute and elsewhere are continuing to enhance Sweden's international reputation in the field of horse medicine.

The three authors of *Keeping your Horse Healthy* are pupils of Forssell, either directly or indirectly. We have had many years of intimate daily contact with practical veterinary treatment of horses. Our book is primarily intended for new horse-owners of all ages; we hope that they will be able to find here all the information that they need to be able to tell when their horses are ill. We have not particularly stressed the importance of calling in the vet when necessary, but this is of course implicit, as is the frequent need for calling him in as quickly as possible, which is mentioned in the text where appropriate.

We hope that this book will be a useful adjunct to the training of grooms, of staff in animal hospitals, of farriers, riders and drivers, and we should be glad to think that some of the information had been useful to the professionals in the world of horse-racing and show-jumping.

Fritz Sevelius
Harry Pettersson
Lennart Olsson

THE SKELETON OF THE HORSE

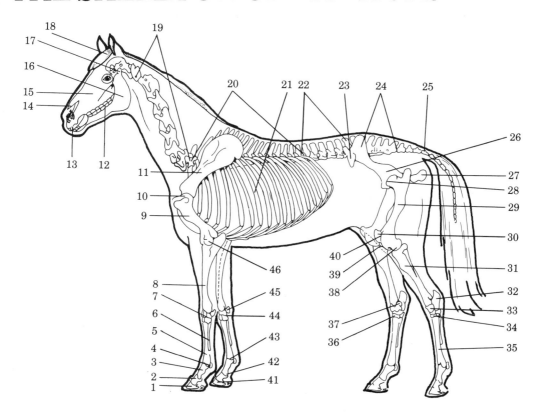

1	Pedal bone	24	5 fused sacral vertebrae
2	Short pastern	25	16 coccygeal vertebrae
3	Long pastern	26	Pelvis
4	Sesamoid bones	27	Ischium
5	Cannon bone or metacarpal	28	Hip joint
6	Splint bone	29	Femur
7	Minor bones of the knee joint	30	Patella
8	Radius	31	Tibia
9	Humerus	32	Hock (Tuber calcis)
10	Shoulder joint	33	Hock (Tarsus)
11	Shoulder blade	34	Hock (Cuboid etc)
12	Cheek teeth	35	Cannon bone or metatarsal
13	Front teeth	36	Hock gliding joints (upper, middle and lower)
14	Nasal bones	37	Hock hinge joint
15	Upper jaw	38	Outer tibial condyle
16	Lower jaw	39	Inner medial condyle
17	Jaw joint	40	Patella or cap and stifle joint
18	Frontal bone	41	Pedal joint
19	7 cervical vertebrae	42	Pastern joint
20	18 thoracic vertebrae	43	Fetlock joint
21	18 ribs	44	Carpus (knee) joints, upper, middle and lower
22	6 lumbar vertebrae	45	Pisiform bone
23	Ilium	46	Elbow joint

VERTICAL SECTION THROUGH THE MIDDLE OF A FORE-FOOT

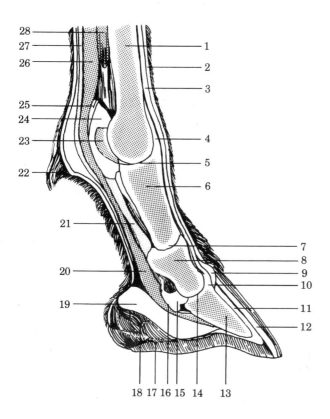

1	Cannon bone or metacarpal
2	Skin
3	Extensor tendon
4	Fetlock joint capsule
5	Fetlock joint
6	Long pastern
7	Pastern joint
8	Short pastern
9	Coronary and perioplic bands
10	Pyramidal structure of pedal bone
11	Horny *laminae*
12	Wall of hoof
13	Pedal bone (coffin bone)
14	Pedal joint
15	Navicular bone
16	Navicular bursa
17	Horny sole
18	Horny frog
19	Fatty frog or plantar cushion
20	Deep flexor tendon
21	Lower part of suspensory ligament
22	Fetlock
23	Sesamoid bones
24	Ligaments of sesamoid bones
25	Great sesamoid tendon sheath
26	Deep flexor tendon
27	Superficial flexor tendon
28	Suspensory ligament

THE MUSCULATURE OF THE HORSE

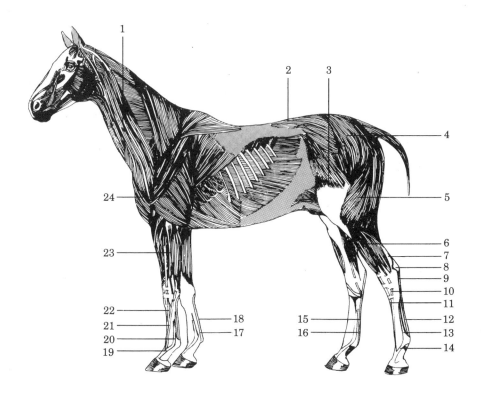

1	Neck muscles	13	Suspensory ligament
2	Extensor muscles of back	14	Check ligaments of suspensory ligament
3	Extensor muscles of stifle	15	Deep flexor tendon
4	Croup muscles	16	Superficial flexor tendon
5	Thigh muscles	17	Deep flexor tendon
6	Leg muscles	18	Superficial flexor tendon
7	Achilles tendon	19	Check ligaments of suspensory ligament
8	Plantar ligament	20	Suspensory ligament
9	Superficial flexor tendon	21	*Extensor suffraginis* tendon
10	*Extensor suffraginis* tendon	22	*Extensor pedis* tendon
11	*Extensor pedis* tendon	23	Muscles of fore-leg
12	Superficial flexor tendon	24	Shoulder muscles

THE INTERNAL ORGANS OF THE HORSE

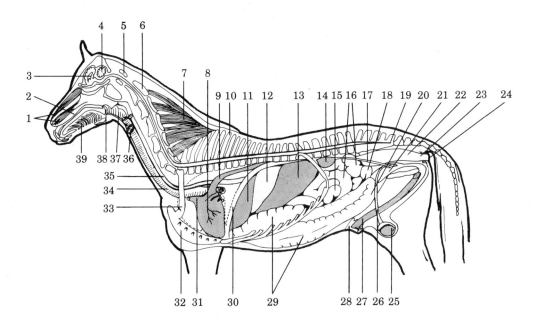

1 False nostrils	21 Bladder
2 Nasal passage	22 Rectum
3 Cerebrum	23 Anal sphincter
4 Cerebellum	24 Anus
5 Atlas, first cervical vertebra	25 Testicle and epididymis
6 Axis, second cervical vertebra	26 Spermatic cord
7 Neck ligaments	27 Penis
8 Heart	28 Sheath
9 Aorta	29 Large intestines (large colon)
10 Spinal processes of thoracic vertebrae	30 Diaphragm
11 Liver	31 Pulmonary artery
12 Stomach	32 Sternum
13 Spleen	33 First rib
14 Kidney	34 Trachea
15 Small intestines	35 Oesophagus
16 Large intestines (small colon)	36 Thyroid gland
17 Urethra	37 Larynx
18 Small intestines	38 Epiglottis
19 Croup bones	39 Tongue
20 Large intestines (pelvic flexure of large colon)	

BREEDING, JUDGING AND STUD-BOOKS

Successful breeding depends entirely upon the correct choice of breeding stock. Different breeds of horse have different characteristics, and it is therefore important to know right from the start what one is trying to achieve, rather than to breed horses at random. In Sweden the importance of setting certain minimum standards was recognised very early on, as was the need for stud-books and for ensuring that the breeding stock actually complied with the standards set.

In 1874 a national horse-registration scheme was introduced, since it was felt to be in the national interest to improve the standard of horse breeding. This scheme is still in operation. The object of the scheme is to register acceptable breeding stock, to enter such horses in the stud-books for their breeds, and to assess their prepotency (ability to transmit their characteristics) by judging their offspring. Grade 'B' is used for an animal entered in a stud-book of its breed, while grade 'A' is used for an animal that has proved its quality as a breed-builder. Formerly there were two categories used to denote grades of prepotency, 'AB' and 'A', but this system was abolished, unfortunately, in 1967.

The inspection of horses for registration is organised by the Swedish Board of Agriculture, which appoints judges for both stallions and mares. Anyone wishing to register a horse has to notify the Board of Agriculture on a special form available from the Board's offices in his county. Applications in the case of a stallion three or more years old should be made by the tenth of January in the year in which the inspection is requested; both application and inspection are free of charge. There is a panel of three judges, one of whom is a veterinary surgeon. Stallions have to reach rather higher standards than mares, because they are likely to have more descendants – some stallions cover 150 mares every year – and can therefore have a greater influence on the development of the breed. This is also the reason why it is illegal to use a stallion for public stud purposes if it is not registered. Even where a number of people share the ownership of such a stallion it is still illegal for any of them to use him for breeding, irrespective of whether any fee is paid.

The inspection of stallions includes examination and evaluation of their pedigree, conformation, soundness, constitution and, depending on the breed, their performance. After being first inspected, a horse may be

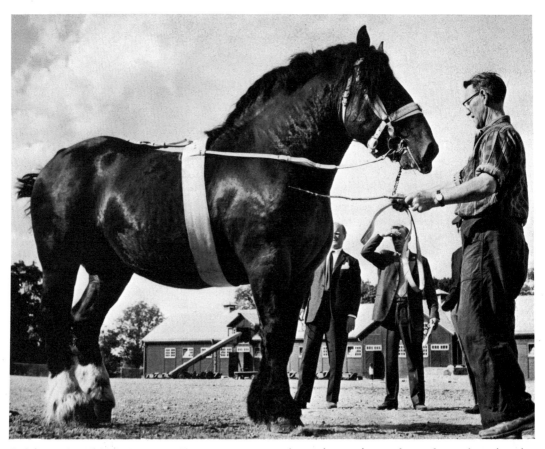

Judging a Swedish Ardennes stallion

allowed to be used for breeding for one year, and this may be extended for a further four years if he passes his second inspection. Older grade 'A' stallions are sometimes allowed to be used for the rest of their lives, but on the other hand a horse that has been passed can subsequently be condemned and removed from the register if his progeny are unsatisfactory. The owner of a stallion that has, in his opinion, been unfairly condemned, has the right of appeal to the Board of Agriculture in the first instance and to the government in the second instance. In the case of stallions of racing breeds (Trotters, English Thoroughbreds) great importance is attached to their performance.

Usually there is a place in each county where inspection takes place, but in the future stallion judging is likely to become more centralised. Mares are inspected during the summer, either at an inspection centre or on their owners' premises. This depends to some extent upon the density of the horse population in particular areas, though here too there is a trend towards centralisation. This is without doubt a good trend, in that it gives less-experienced horse-owners a chance to compare their horses with others, and thus counteracts their natural tendency to see only the good points of their own horses. Mares are not judged by such stringent standards as stallions, and usually only pedigree, conformation, disposition and the quality of their foals are taken into account. A mare must have a foal running with her to be eligible for registration, and the foal

16

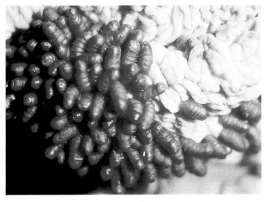

Botfly, *Gasterophilus intestinalis.* Larvae and pupae attached to the mucous membranes of the stomach wall

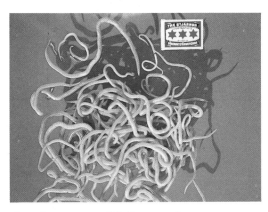

Ascaris equorum. Adult worms from six-month-old foal

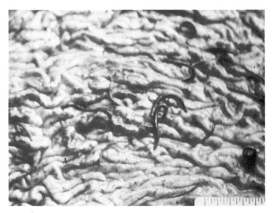

Redworms, *Strongylus vulgaris.* Adult worms attached to intestinal mucous membranes

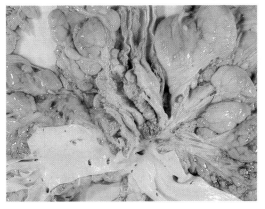

Redworm larvae attached to the wall of the aorta

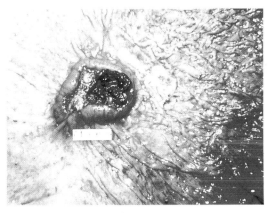

Small redworms (*Strongylus*). The picture shows damage to the mucous membrane caused by the entry of the larvae. This can lead to secondary infections

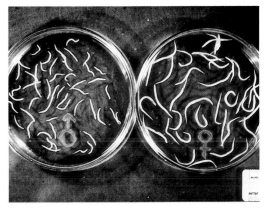

Seatworms, *Oxyuris.* Adult worms, male (♂), female (♀)

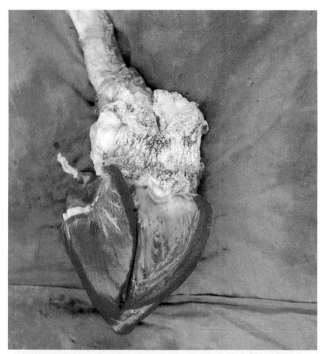

Damage to the wall of an artery and heart valves, caused by redworm larvae

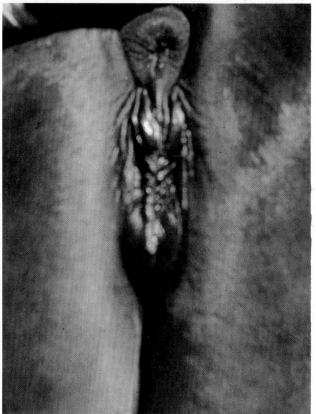

Mare with coital exanthema

must be by a registered stallion of the same breed.

Since 1967 both stallions and mares must pass a working trial. Ponies and blood horses may be either driven or ridden, cold-blooded horses must be driven. Trotters must reach certain minimum standards of performance, while standards set for half-blood stallions are more stringent.

Successful breed improvement is impossible if the choice of animals from which to breed is too limited. Sweden is a small country with relatively few horses, and it has always been necessary to limit the numbers of breeds that are recognised, in the interest of improving the quality of these breeds. Twenty years ago the number of recognised breeds was very small, but a recent relaxation of import restrictions and an increased international contact has led to a great increase in the number of breeds recognised by the Board of Agriculture. In 1976 these breeds were:

Blood horses: English, Arabian and Anglo-Arabian, Arabian half-bred, Swedish warm-blood and thoroughbred Trotter.

Ponies: Gotland, Shetland, Welsh Mountain, Welsh, New Forest, Connemara.

Cold-blooded horses: Fjord horse, North Swedish trotter, North-Swedish draught horse, Swedish Ardennes horse.

Judging ponies

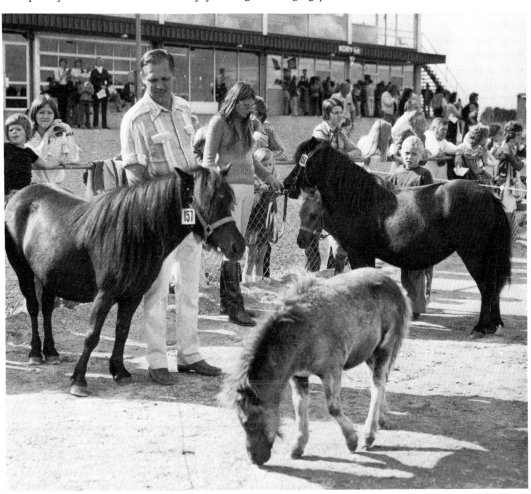

To be eligible for registration a horse must have a pedigree traceable to the appropriate Swedish or recognised foreign stud-books.

Some breeding of horses not listed above does go on in Sweden – for example, Iceland horses, Exmoor ponies and Lippizaner horses. There are no stud-books for these breeds in Sweden, but nevertheless the stallions must be inspected in the normal way before being used, although the mares are exempt. Cross-bred horses are not inspected, and cross-bred stallions may not be used for breeding.

Inspection of foals of recognised breeds takes place when the mares are being inspected; one-, two- and three-year-old mares and sometimes stallions are shown, and are judged for conformation only. Some breed societies offer certificates and prize money, but strictly speaking this is outside the registration scheme. Applications to have young horses inspected are made at the same time as for fully-grown horses.

Older registered horses can also be awarded the higher grade, 'A'. A mare qualifies by producing four good foals, two of which are passed for registration. As usual, stallions have to pass more stringent tests; to qualify, they must produce ten or more descendants four or more years old, which are either registered or otherwise of proven quality.

For stallions of racing breeds an even larger number of comparable offspring is required.

Compulsory registration of stallions, and the whole horse-inspection scheme, have been of fundamental importance to Swedish horse-breeding, and are responsible for the high international reputation of Swedish horses. That the system has been continuously in operation for over 100 years is also widely recognised as a sign of stability.

The registration scheme prevents the use of inferior stallions, and ensures that only mares that meet minimum requirements are used for breeding. The authorities are well aware that these measures have effectively protected the Swedish breeds from deterioration which could have been caused by the recent careless importation of poor-quality horses by less responsible importers.

There were approximately 102,000 horses in Sweden in 1975, of which there were 42,000 Thoroughbreds, 17,000 ponies, 28,000 cold-blooded horses, and 15,000 horses of less specific types, mainly Thoroughbred in character.

The most common breed is the Swedish warm-blood (22,000), followed by thorough-bred Trotters (16,500) and Swedish Ardennes (11,000). The commonest pony is the Gotland, with approximately 8,000.

THE GYNAECOLOGY OF THE MARE

THE ANATOMY OF THE MARE'S REPRODUCTIVE ORGANS

The ovaries consist of several thousand follicles each containing an ovum or egg. These follicles, which are present prior to the mare's birth, are too small to be seen by the naked eye. Each ovary joins the rather funnel-shaped mouth of one of the fallopian tubes, which contain thousands of fine, flexible cilia which propel the egg down towards

The mare's reproductive organs

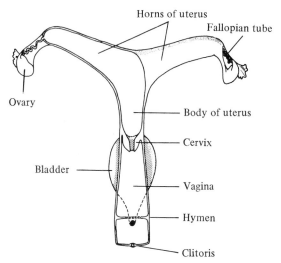

the womb. Fertilisation always takes place in one of the fallopian tubes.

The foetus develops in the womb or uterus. The inner layer (the endometrium) is like soft velvet, and it is from this layer that oxygen and nutrients are transferred from the mare to her foal. The endometrium is regulated by means of hormones.

The mouth of the womb (the cervix) opens or closes the passage from the vagina into the womb. It is usually completely closed, especially during pregnancy, but during heat (oestrus) the cervix relaxes, opens and allows the sperm to enter the womb. Mares come on heat at intervals throughout a breeding season which lasts from February or March to September or October. Individual mares can often vary considerably from the norm, and it is difficult to differentiate between normal and abnormal oestrous cycles.

THE OESTRUS CYCLE

The oestrous cycle is regulated by large numbers of different sex hormones. A hormone is a special substance which is produced in an organ or tissue and which, after being transported by either blood or lymph to an entirely different organ elsewhere in the body, is able to produce there certain specific reactions.

21

The main source of sex hormones is the pituitary, a small gland which lies just below the brain, but the ovaries, the womb and the testicles also produce such hormones. The pituitary is regulated by certain centres within the brain.

During the winter the pituitary produces relatively few sex hormones, but in the spring the rise in temperature and the increased hours of both sunshine and daylight, often coupled with more or better food such as lush new grass, stimulate the brain into increasing the production of sex hormones in the pituitary. This activates the reproductive organs, and the mare's oestrous cycle begins.

We know very little about the mechanism which causes a particular follicle in the ovary to be chosen from the thousands present, and to grow rapidly, reaching a diameter of up to 60mm when ripe. The growing follicle has great though short-lived powers of hormone production, its innermost layer producing large quantities of oestrogen, a hormone which is carried to the brain by the bloodstream and triggers off all the visible symptoms of heat or oestrus. Oestrogen also influences the womb, the cervix and the vagina; circulation to these organs increases, and as a result large quantities of mucus are produced in the womb and vagina. This mucus assists the passage of the stallion's sperm in the womb and the fallopian tubes.

A complex hormonal stimulus causes the follicle to rupture and to empty its contents slowly into the fallopian tube (ovulation). Mares coming on heat early in the year (February–March) often have difficulty ovulating, sometimes staying on heat for several weeks without the follicle rupturing. This is caused by a hormonal deficiency, and the best treatment is probably to wait for nature to take its course and to mate the mare later at the more normal season (April–May–June). This is particularly common in young mares.

The empty follicle rapidly fills with blood, and can easily be felt during a *per rectum* examination. The mare reacts to palpation of the blood-filled follicle with obvious symptoms of pain. The innermost layer of cells in the follicle grows rapidly, and the blood is replaced by cells which produce special hormones. This is a yellow body (*corpus luteum*), a temporary but important gland which produces the hormone progesterone.

Progesterone is antagonistic towards oestrogen. Increasing amounts of progesterone in the bloodstream quickly put an end to the oestrous stage of the cycle. The yellow body produces large quantities of progesterone for the next fourteen days, and then begins to be re-absorbed. As the amount of progesterone in the blood decreases, the pituitary gland is released from the inhibiting effect of progesterone, and resumes its production of sex hormones, leading to the mare coming on heat once more.

OESTRUS

The equine reproductive system differs in many ways from those of other domesticated animals. Thus the mare comes on heat only about nine days after giving birth, though this can vary somewhat. Sometimes the 'foal heat' comes only five or six days after birth, sometimes after fifteen or sixteen days. The length of the whole oestrous cycle, ie the period between the first day of heat in one cycle and the first day of heat in the next, is usually given as twenty-one days (three weeks). Here too there can be considerable variation, and a mare's owner should study her behaviour patterns so as to discover how long she stays on heat and the length of her whole cycle.

Diagnosing oestrus. It is often difficult to tell if a mare is on heat or not. The best way to

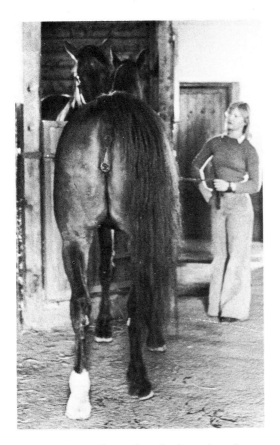

The mare here shows that she is on heat by lifting her tail when being 'teased'

mare's genitalia; infections, bleeding and sores can easily be seen. The vet can also examine a mare by rectal palpation, feeling the uterus and the ovaries. If a follicle is ready to rupture this can be felt, and often the vet can estimate the most suitable time to cover (mate) the mare by feeling the consistency of the follicle.

COVERING

Mares are often covered at the 'foal heat' which is about nine days after giving birth. In such cases mares should be carefully examined by a vet. Often the womb will not have returned to its normal size, and any damage to the birth canal will not have healed completely. Covering at the foal heat

A partition protects the stallion from being kicked if the mare is not yet, or no longer, on heat

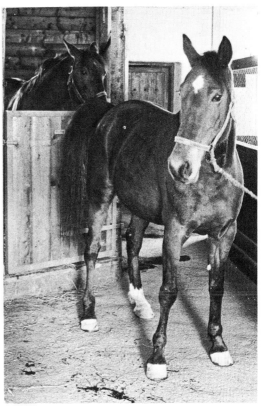

find out is by 'teasing' her. If she is led to a stallion, she will show certain typical symptoms if she is on heat, such as lifting her tail, putting her hind-quarters in a receptive posture, 'winking' her vulva and, in so doing, showing a clear mucous discharge. When being teased a mare should always be hobbled to prevent her from kicking the stallion, or she can be led to the other side of a partition of some sort, such as the door of the stallion's stall, as in the photographs pp 23–6.

If there is still any doubt, a vet can soon settle the matter by inspecting the mare with a vaginal speculum. It is then possible to see the relaxed cervix, the redness of the mucosa, etc. Such an examination will also give a good indication of the general health of the

23

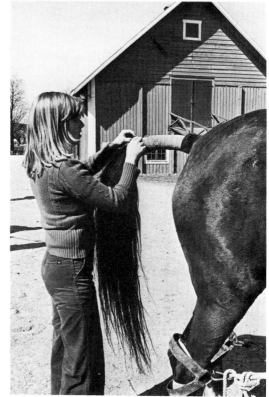

(right) The mare's tail is bandaged before covering, and she is hobbled to prevent her kicking the stallion

(below) The stallion is led up to the mare

(opposite above) When the stallion mounts the mare her tail should be drawn aside

(opposite below) The stallion ejaculating

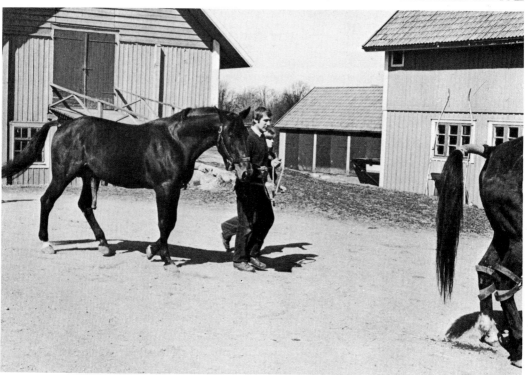

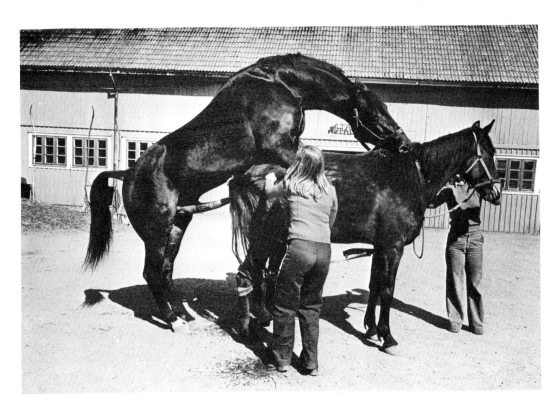

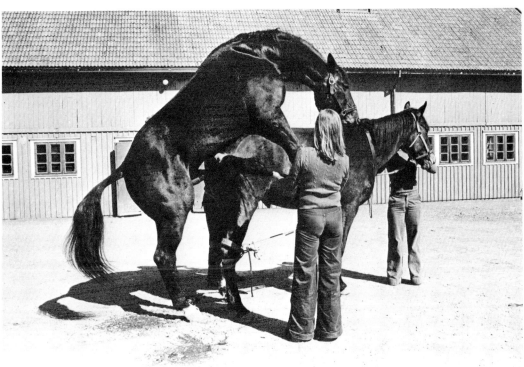

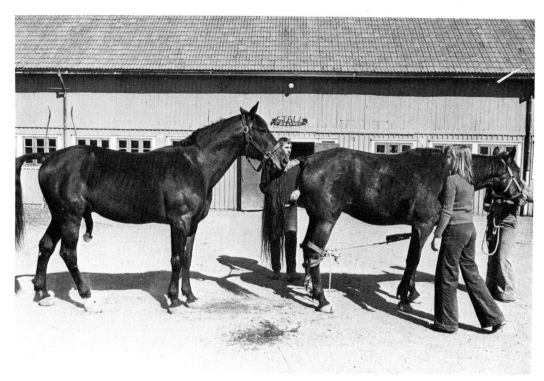

Covering is over

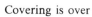

The mare's oestrus is over and she is no longer interested in the stallion

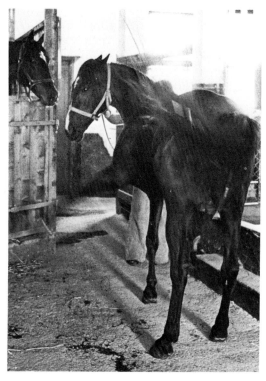

should be avoided whenever possible, and a mare that has just had her first foal should never be covered at this heat.

Choose a secluded spot for covering, where the ground is firm and neither slippery nor dusty. The mare should be hobbled, the root of her tail should be bandaged and her vulva cleaned with a mild and preferably odourless antiseptic solution. The stallion's penis should be inspected before and after covering, and afterwards it should be washed with an antiseptic that will not cause irritation. Covering is usually repeated every other day (ie at 48-hour intervals) as long as the mare stays on heat.

Too frequent covering can increase the risk of an infection of the uterus. Mares should be covered as infrequently as possible, which can be partly achieved by increasing the interval to 2½–3 days. The sperm lives and is fully fertile for at least three days in the fallopian tubes, which is where fertilisation occurs.

Ideally a mare should mate only once during the oestrous period. If a vet examines the ovaries and the development of the follicle he can often advise the owner as to the best time to mate the mare, thus lessening the risk of infection.

The best time for a mare to be covered is about twenty-four hours before ovulation. It is very difficult to determine when the follicle will rupture, but an experienced vet will usually give valuable advice. Oestrus ends about twenty-four hours after ovulation, and fertilisation rarely takes place when a mare is covered after ovulation.

After ovulation and for twenty-four hours thereafter the mare often behaves characteristically if attempts are made to cover her, moving her tail from side to side, shifting her weight irritably from one hind leg to the other, and making a high-pitched whinny.

If the mare has been covered and, with luck, has also ovulated, one or sometimes two eggs starting their journey down to the womb, certain changes soon occur in the vulval area. The vulval lips become smaller and close tightly together, and a milky deposit is often seen on the skin below the vulva. Try to find out as soon as possible if the mare has become pregnant. This may be done by 'teasing' her at 14–15 days after she was last covered, and again every 2 or 3 days until the 25th or 26th day.

If you suspect that she may be on heat again, the vet should be called in to examine her.

Some pregnant mares show indistinct signs of heat for a short time around the 21st day. These mares can be covered with some difficulty, and there is considerable risk of abortion.

PREGNANCY EXAMINATION

An experienced vet performing a *per rectum* examination at 20–22 days can usually be fairly certain whether a mare is pregnant or not.

Normally a mare is examined *per rectum* at 40–42 days. The advantage of an examination at this stage is that the vet can tell immediately whether the mare is pregnant or not, and if she is not pregnant he can tell her owner about her general gynaecological condition, eg onset of oestrus, follicle development, infections.

There are other ways of finding out whether a mare is pregnant. A blood test is a very reliable method; a blood sample is taken by a vet and sent for analysis between the 49th and the 70th day. At 4 months or later the urine can be tested chemically to determine whether a mare is pregnant.

If a mare becomes pregnant after having been covered early in the season (February–March) it is wise to examine her before the end of the season. In 8–10 per cent of pregnancies the foetus dies at some time between the 20th and the 90th day, and is resorbed or aborted. In such cases the vet can induce the mare to come into heat again, so that she may still become pregnant in that season.

Never examine a mare that may be pregnant between the 30th and the 39th day. At this time complex cell movements are taking place in the womb, controlled by complex hormonal stimuli. Pregnant mares should be kept as quiet and free from stress as possible at this stage. Don't change their fodder or change their routine, and avoid veterinary treatment if possible; in other words, let them lead as normal and stress-free an existence as possible.

CAUSES OF STERILITY

Only 60–70 per cent of mated mares become pregnant. There are various reasons for this, but it is often because mares are mated at the wrong time of year or at the wrong time during oestrus.

Defective hormone production. It is rare for a mare to become pregnant if she is covered just before shedding her winter coat, when she is in poor condition, lacking vitamins and without sufficient vitality for the reproductive organs to function properly. Mares may well come into heat, but the symptoms will be weak and the oestrous period will drag on without ovulation taking place. This is most common in racehorses that have been raced or trained hard recently.

This condition is caused by the pituitary gland producing enough hormones early in the spring to stimulate follicle development to partial ripeness, while production of the luteinising hormone which causes the rupture of the follicle is still quite inadequate, so that ovulation is not possible. Mares in general produce small quantities of the luteinising

hormone relative to other animals, which is why their oestrous period is comparatively long. These partially ripe follicles can sometimes be stimulated into ovulating by the injection of luteinising hormones (chorionic gonadotrophin).

Cysts. Ovarian cysts are rare, and so-called cysts are often follicles which have failed to ovulate and remain in an arrested stage of development. Often these disappear during the winter. If a true cyst is diagnosed, the cyst and the entire ovary should be removed surgically as soon as possible, for most ovarian cysts can be the early stages of tumours. Mares with only one ovary can still breed, and there are many examples of such mares that have had several foals.

Infections of the uterus. Infections in the womb are a common cause of sterility. Most mares become infected during mating or while giving birth, but it is also possible for a general infection to become localised in the uterus.

Systematic bacteriological examinations of mares have demonstrated that 100 per cent suffer from infection on the first day after giving birth. This percentage falls until in a normal sample only 20–25 per cent are infected at the foal heat nine days after foaling. This is a convincing argument against the practice of covering mares at the foal heat. If this practice could be eradicated the incidence of infected mares could be reduced considerably.

Another cause of infection is having mares covered at too short intervals. A popular stallion may be used too much, perhaps covering mares 3–5 times a day, which does not permit his sexual organ to cleanse and heal itself. Thus he can be an agent in the transmission of infection from infected to uninfected mares.

Most infections of the uterus can be demonstrated to have been caused by streptococci bacteria, but staphylococci, coli, and even fungi are sometimes found. Viruses will almost certainly also be present in infected mares.

Treatment of inflammation of the uterus is difficult and time-consuming. It is rarely responsive to a single irrigation of the womb with antibiotics. Usually it is necessary to find out which type of bacteria is causing the infection and to test the reaction of the bacteria to various antibiotics in the laboratory. Then the mare is treated both locally and generally with the appropriate antibiotics until she can be given a bacteriological test at her next oestrus. *A bacteriological test is only reliable if it is carried out while the mare is in oestrus.*

Often mares will be found to suffer from different types of infection at each oestrus, and in such cases one is entitled to assume that the mucous membrane lining the womb has lost its natural resistance to infection. Such mares are very difficult to cure, and often show little response to treatment.

Windsucking. Vaginal windsucking is commonest in Thoroughbred horses, Arabians and other blood-horses. The vulval lips are slack, particularly during oestrus, and do not close very closely, thus permitting air to be sucked into the vagina when the horse moves, causing the vagina to become blown up like a balloon.

The air sucked in will generally contain micro-organisms, particularly those found in the dung (*E. coli*). During oestrus the cervix is generally wide open, allowing the infected air to enter the womb and cause a serious infection. Treatment is to operate, stitching together the lips which form the upper part of the vulva (Caslick operation).

Note that such mares will burst these stitches when they foal, so they should be re-stitched immediately afterwards. It is good practice to cut the mare at the site of the Caslick operation before the foal is born, thus easing delivery and the subsequent re-stitching.

Coital exanthema is caused by a virus belonging to the herpes group. Both stallions and mares are affected, and the virus may be transmitted in either direction during mating. Small blisters or vessicles appear on the mare's vulva, which burst leaving ulcerated areas which quickly heal. If damage has been caused at any depth in the skin or mucous membrane the pigmentation is usually damaged, leaving white scars where the sores have healed. Stallions also develop these vessicles on both penis and prepuce. Infected horses may run a temperature or go off their food. Stallions are infected by mares that have this disease and pass it on to other mares.

Neither stallions nor mares with coital exanthema should be allowed to mate until the sores have healed.

The sores usually heal within 10–20 days.

Coital exanthema in a stallion

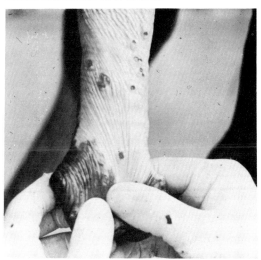

Antibiotics are used to prevent secondary infections, and are administered both locally and generally.

It should be stressed here that this disease does *not* cause infertility, but it can considerably disrupt the schedule of a busy stallion.

ABORTION

In Sweden 8–10 per cent of pregnancies end with the death of the foetus between the 20th and the 90th day; expulsion of the foetus (abortion) is rare, it being more usual for the placenta and the foetus to be reabsorbed. If the foetus dies after 38 days or more the mare continues to produce certain sex hormones which prevent her from coming into heat for 3–4 months.

Causes can range from deficient progesterone production to neglected uterine infections which spread until the toxins damage the foetus. It is also believed that inherited deformities in the foetus may be a possible cause, and that this is nature's way of preventing the birth of abnormal individuals.

Spontaneous abortion. Sometimes mares abort during the autumn or winter. There may be several reasons for this. Sometimes it can be shown that the foetus was suffering from a bacterial infection, but more usually bacteriological and virological examinations are negative and the abortion is put down to a hormonal imbalance.

Viral abortion. See Infectious Diseases, p 67.

In spite of the efforts of owners, stallion leaders, veterinary surgeons and others, only two-thirds of all mated mares conceive, for a variety of reasons. Owners tend to forget these barren mares until the spring, when their enthusiasm is rekindled and they suddenly become keen to mate them again. Many of these mares are suffering from conditions which rule out conception; they may have ovarian cysts, uterine infections or obstructed cervices, or they may be wind-suckers.

Often these conditions are difficult to cure, and it is best to examine all barren mares during the autumn or winter to allow plenty of time for restoring them to health before mating them in the spring.

THE PREGNANT MARE

Pregnant mares should be allowed to live a normal life with a reasonable amount of exercise every day. They should not be expected to do any very strenuous types of training, but being judicially ridden or driven every day will do nothing but good.

Two-thirds of the growth of the foetus takes place during the last third of the pregnancy, and a mare's owner should be particularly careful to ensure that her ration then contains sufficient calories, minerals, vitamins etc. Never let pregnant mares get fat; a mare without too much fat and with well exercised muscles will be better able to deliver a more healthy foal.

The gestation period can vary considerably. It is normally said to be 11 months, but many mares produce small but often perfectly healthy foals after only 10 months, while others exceed the normal gestation period. There are plenty of cases on record of mares giving birth to large but perfectly normal foals after being pregnant for more than a year.

BIRTH

There are many signs that a mare is about to foal. The first is that the udder starts to swell. This may first be noticed about a month before the mare is due to foal, and

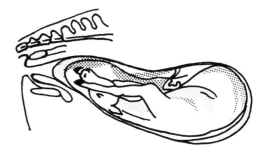

Normal foetal position

should be watched in case one half of the udder becomes swollen too quickly and gets very hard, which is a sign of mastitis. Between the halves of the udder a dark brown ointment-like secretion often collects, produced by glands in the skin of the udder. This secretion often contains a lot of bacteria; the udder, especially the division between the halves, should be washed very carefully 2–3 days before the mare foals. The udder should then be carefully rinsed with clean water to remove any smell or taste which might be offputting to the newborn foal.

Another sign is the relaxation of the mare's pelvis as the result of a slackening of the tension in the ligaments which limit the size of the aperture in the pelvis through which the birth canal passes. An increase in

31

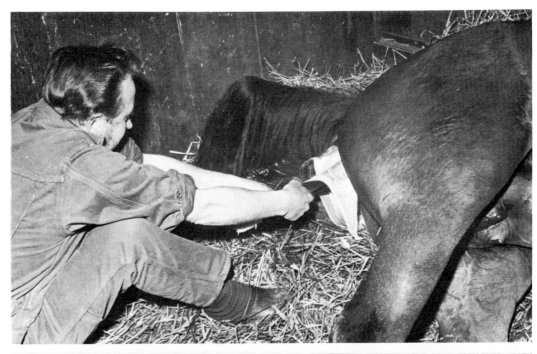

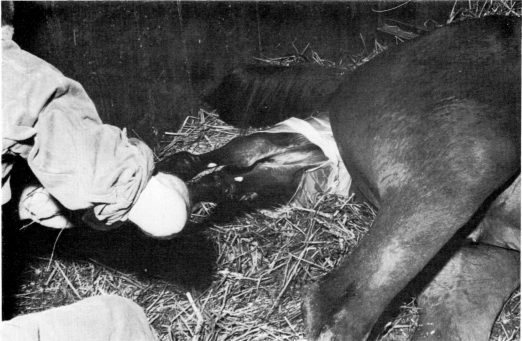

Birth in progress. The attendant is pulling
carefully in time with the mare's contractions

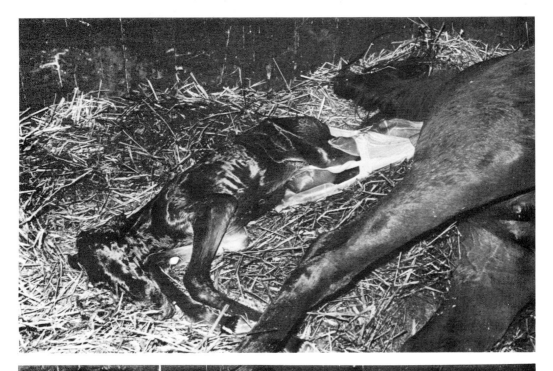

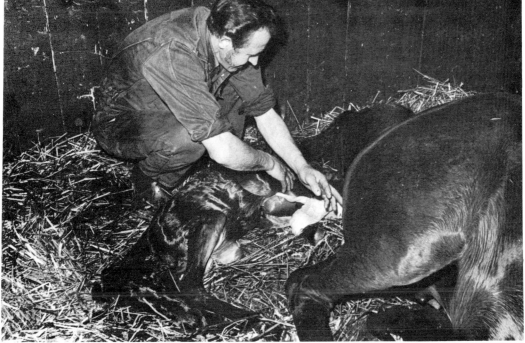

The foal is born and the umbilical cord is still intact

When the pulsation has stopped the umbilical cord is tied off with a sterile bandage if it bleeds

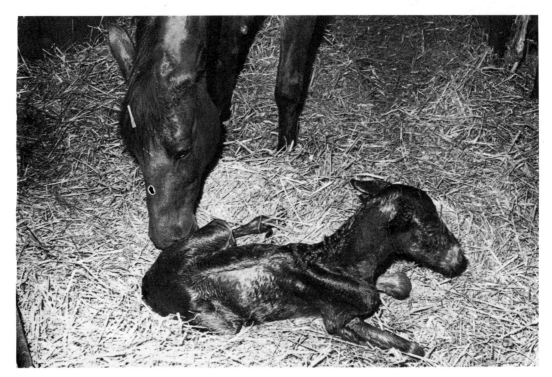

The mare licks her foal dry. The tongue
massages the foal's abdomen, stimulating the
foal to void the meconium

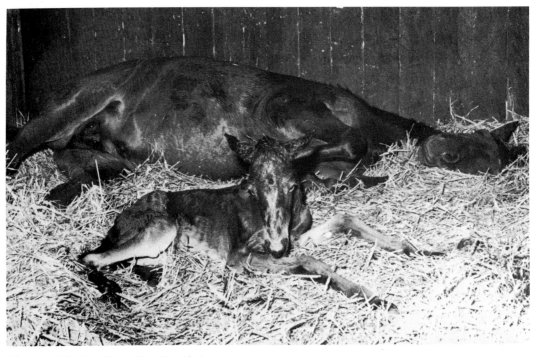

Mare and foal resting after the birth

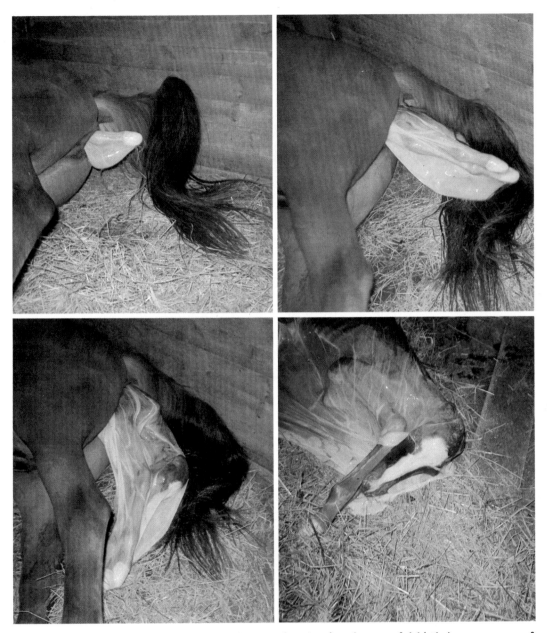

A natural and successful birth in a sequence of eight photographs

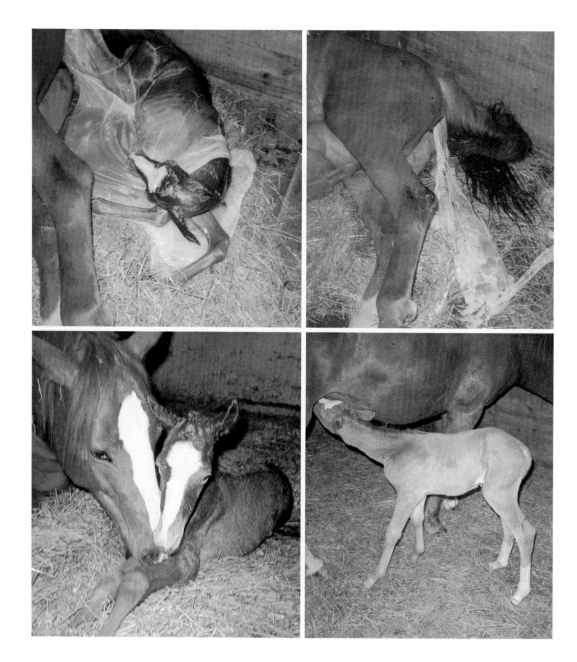

the supply of blood and lymph to the sheaths surrounding these ligaments gives them greater elasticity than normal, so that at birth they will stretch and give a wider passage for the foal. This relaxation begins near the root of the tail, spreading towards the croup, and is complete by the time birth starts. It is most easily noticed in mares with wide, flat, well developed croups.

Two or three days before foaling some mares start to behave very peculiarly, walking round and round in the loose-box, often making a distinct circular track, and stopping from time to time to throw up their heads and stare absently ahead. They then continue walking round, the whole phase lasting for 6–8 hours, after which their behaviour returns to normal. Possibly this phase marks the movement of the foal in the womb to the normal pre-birth position.

One very reliable sign that a mare is about to foal is what is known as 'waxing up'. A drop of 'wax' – actually the protein-rich colostrum which precedes the flow of milk – is forced from each teat and coagulates in the air. This is reliable in older mares but less so in mares foaling for the first time, since their udders are usually small and underdeveloped and cannot retain milk properly.

A foaling box should be prepared well in advance. It should be very clean with a soft, firm floor strewn with plenty of clean, long straw, free from dust. Never use chaff or short, broken straw in a foaling box. Lay plenty of straw along the walls and especially in the corners.

If the foaling box is to be used by several mares it must be cleaned extremely thoroughly after each birth, as an infected foaling box becomes an ideal breeding ground for deadly foal infections.

Immediately before she starts to foal a mare often begins to sweat on the sides of the neck and behind the elbows on the sides of the chest. Mares give birth quickly; the process is controlled by hormones, and the contractions of both the uterus and the muscles of the wall of the abdomen are very powerful. The mare's pelvis is also such that the foal can easily pass through it.

Birth usually takes about 15 minutes, from the first appearance of the amnion to the completed birth of the foal. Most mares can normally foal unassisted, but an experienced attendant should always be at hand. It is best to be as quiet and unobtrusive as possible; ideally, the mare should not be aware that she is being observed, particularly in the early stages.

Some mares, particularly older mares or mares that have never foaled before, may need a little help. Pull in the right direction, in a curve down towards the points of the mare's hocks, in time with the mare's contractions. Avoid pulling too hard or too jerkily!

If the birth is in any way delayed or complicated, the experienced attendant, having very carefully washed his hands and arms, may try to alter the position of the foal in the birth canal. In fairly simple cases, such as when a fore-leg is bent slightly backwards, the attendant should quickly be able to put everything to rights, probably saving the foal's life.

An inexperienced attendant should only try to locate and correct a wrong position or presentation if there is no possibility of getting the help of a vet or an experienced attendant; he should be very careful, and it is essential that he should know the correct birth position for the foal. If the presentation is seriously wrong the vet must be called *immediately*, but often the owner must resign himself to the likelihood of the foal dying before anything can be done.

When the head and neck are free the

mucus and the amnion (foetal membrane) should be cleared away from around the foal's nostrils. It is best to allow the hind-legs to remain partially in the birth canal; this gives the mare some contact with her foal, so that she lies quietly and the umbilical cord is not severed prematurely. The umbilical cord, the link between the mare and her foal, through which the foetus is nourished, will now be stretched between the foal's abdomen and the placenta, which is still in the mare's womb. If one pinches the cord with one's fingers a strong pulse can be felt. After birth 0.5–1.5 litres of blood are pumped through the umbilical cord from the mare to her foal. This blood transfusion is vital for the new-born foal, so be very careful with the umbilical cord and do not let it be severed until these pulsations have ceased (approx. 10–15 minutes).

When the pulsations have stopped it is time to break this connection between the mare and the foal. Usually the cord ruptures naturally when the mare moves her hind-quarters or stands up. If one examines the umbilical cord, a slight thinness or weakening may be noticed about 3–5cm from the foal's abdomen, which is where it should be broken. If you break it yourself, you should place one hand on the foal's abdomen to support the navel while pulling and twisting the cord with the other hand. If the cord is pulled strongly without the navel being supported the membranes and muscles of the abdomen can easily be damaged, which may lead to an umbilical hernia. When the cord has broken it should be treated with an antiseptic preparation – such as tincture of iodine – which must have the effect of contracting and drying out the cord, so that the blood vessels are quickly sealed off.

If there is much bleeding from the navel, which is particularly common in the Swedish Ardennes breed or other heavy horse breeds, the navel should be tied off to prevent loss of blood.

Cleanliness is vital! Boil all sutures and ligatures to sterilise them, and clean the umbilical cord carefully. A special bandage may be used, or linen tape like that used to make loops on towels, or in an emergency a gauze bandage. The ligature should be left in place for 1–2 days. It is very easy to seal in an infection which then spreads up the blood vessels to the liver, causing a general infection which may kill the foal.

The afterbirth should be passed naturally within ½–3 hours after the birth. Spread it out on the floor to make sure that it has all been passed; look for the innermost horn-shaped parts. If the afterbirth is retained, take the mare away from the foal for 10–15 minutes every hour and lead her, run with her or put her in a paddock. Being separated from her foal will make her very uneasy; she will neigh, kick and strain, so that her muscles will bear down upon the womb, helping it to contract and speeding up the passing of the afterbirth. If fairly vigorous exercise does not do the trick within 12 hours, the vet should be called.

A mare that has just foaled should in any case be separated from her foal for 15–30 minutes at least once a day. The anxiety she then feels about her foal makes her very active, which helps the contraction, cleansing and healing of the birth canal. This is particularly beneficial if the mare's owner wishes to mate the mare at the 'foal heat' about nine days after the birth of the foal. Many mares also produce more milk as a result of this exercise.

THE NEWLY BORN AND GROWING FOAL

A new-born foal should start trying to stand about an hour after birth, and should soon try to take its first hesitant and wobbly steps.

Foals often find it difficult to balance their hind-quarters. If a foal is helped to its feet too soon it often overbalances; its hind-quarters may collapse and it can easily fall over backwards and give its head and neck a nasty blow on the floor or the wall. If a foal is weak and fails to stand after several attempts, it may help to give it its first feed from a bottle. Remember that the teat must be clean and all bottles and containers sterilised. An intravenous injection of B vitamins often helps. If the foal still cannot stand after six hours the vet should be consulted.

When the foal is on its feet and has taken a few steps its instinct soon prompts it to search for its mother's udder. Most foals quickly find the teats, and there is no finer sound than the gurgling as they swallow their first milk.

Sometimes a foal may have difficulty in finding the teats and suckling. It takes a lot of time and patience to teach such a foal; it is no good trying to push its neck down to get its head near the udder, as this only seems to make it more obstinately determined to stick its head and neck up in the air! The best method usually is to guide the foal's hind-quarters so that its head approaches the mare, and to guide the teats in the direction of its mouth from the other side of the mare.

Some foals find difficulty in locating the udder because of poorly developed reflexes, and there is a limit to the length of time that such foals can go without food. Any artificial feeding of the mare's milk to foals like these must be regulated so that the foal is always thirsty and hungry, but still has enough energy to continue to look for its mother's udder.

The foal is given a little help to stand up and start suckling. This must be done very carefully, in case the foal falls over and hurts itself

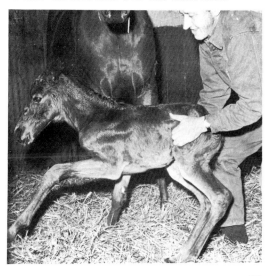

FEEDING FOALS ARTIFICIALLY

Sometimes a mare may die during foaling, having given birth to a live foal. In other cases a mare may refuse to accept her foal, or may be unable to produce milk.

In such cases artificial feeding is necessary. If possible the foal should be given colostrum, the milk which is produced during the first twelve hours after birth.

It is a good plan, at least on larger stud-farms, to keep a supply of frozen colostrum (a colostrum bank) in the freezer, so that a motherless new-born foal can be given as good a start in life as possible. It is also easy to 'steal' 20–30cl from any normal quiet mares that have just foaled. The best way to rear an orphaned foal is to find it a foster mother, but this is not always easy; there are cases on record of foals having been fostered by cows or goats, but in general the only solution is to feed the foal artificially. Cows' milk is often used as a substitute for mares' milk, but it is not suitable, being very different in composition. Cows' milk contains much more fat than mares' milk, while mares' milk contains more milk sugar (lactose).

It is better to use a preparatory milk substitute, made up according to the instructions either of the vet or of the manufacturers. It is important to do this as cleanly and hygienically as possible, to sterilise all utensils (teats, bottles, receptacles) before use and to dispose of any milk substitute that may be left over. The temperature of the mixture should be 37–40°C. For the first few days it may be necessary to use a feeding bottle with a teat, but this is a very time-consuming method, and the foal should be taught to drink from a bowl as soon as possible.

The amount of fluid that a foal requires depends upon its size. A new-born hot-blooded foal weighs approximately 50kg, and normally doubles its birth weight at around two months old. The daily fluid requirement is about 1 litre per 10kg body weight. Thus a newly born foal needs about 5 litres of fluid every twenty-four hours, increasing according to the speed at which the foal grows.

How often, and how much, should a foal be fed?

A normal foal, during the first few days after birth, suckles about every half-hour, drinking 20–30cl each time. The ideal when feeding artificially is to copy nature as closely as possible. Small quantities should be fed at as frequent intervals as possible, and in all cases no less frequently than eight times every twenty-four hours.

As the foal grows older the quantity given at each feed may be increased and the feeds may be given at less frequent intervals.

A foal 2–3 months old should consume up to 15–17 litres of milk substitute every twenty-four hours. The most common error when feeding artificially is to give foals too much nourishment and too little fluid, so that they often become too fat. It is important that these orphan foals should be given the opportunity to learn to eat hay and concentrates with mineral supplements as soon as possible, so that the troublesome period during which they are artificially fed may be as short as possible. It is also important for orphan foals to get plenty of exercise, so that normal bowel function is maintained.

Motherless foals are very susceptible to infections, and should be frequently examined by the vet.

MECONIUM RETENTION

A new-born foal's rectum and intestines normally contain hard, dark pellets of dung (meconium) which are normally voided some 6–12 hours after birth. The first milk (colostrum) contains laxative substances which increase bowel activity and speed up the passing of the meconium. Some foals have difficulty in passing it, particularly small foals with narrow pelvic girdles.

The symptoms of meconium retention are quite dramatic. The foal shows all the symptoms of severe colic and can make extraordinary contortions. Often foals may have cramp in the small intestine as well. The treatment is to rid the foal of these hard pellets; often a laxative jelly introduced into the end of the rectum (*ampulla recti*) does the trick, and using well lubricated rubber gloves it may be possible to remove the pellets just inside the anal sphincter. Sometimes an enema may be necessary, and occasionally surgery is the only cure. The surest sign that the blockage has been removed is a sudden improvement in the foal's condition; often it will suckle normally and for long periods and pass the yellow milk dung, which has a creamy consistency and is often mixed with bubbles of gas.

WET TAIL

Normally most foals suffer from a form of diarrhoea ('wet tail') at the time of the mare's 'foal heat', which is caused by certain hormonal changes affecting the mare's milk. The area around the foal's anus becomes badly soiled and the foal may develop a nervous habit of moving the tail from side to side, rubbing the faeces into the skin and causing irritation and loss of hair. This can be avoided if the skin is cleaned with a little warm water and protected by a layer of liquid paraffin. This diarrhoea should normally cease when the mare goes off heat.

In foals diarrhoea with other causes can often be very serious, especially if the foal's general condition deteriorates as a result of loss of appetite and dehydration caused by the diarrhoea. The vet should be called at once if signs of dehydration are seen.

INFECTIONS

General infections in foals can be very dangerous. During the first year of life a foal has very low resistance to infections. Little natural resistance has been built up, and the lining of the intestines is incapable of hindering the passage of bacteria, viruses and antigens during the first few days of life. Infections can enter via the stomach and the intestines, via the navel and via the respiratory tract.

A common pattern is for small premature foals to be infected by a strain of the shigella group with a very high resistance to antibiotics. At first the foal suffering from 'sleepy foal disease' is very lively, resting little and often walking in an inquisitive and nervous way round the loose-box. It suckles rarely, and for very short periods, and after 6–12 hours it lies down and sinks gradually into lethargy, apathy and unconsciousness, usually dying within 12–24 hours of the onset of the disease. If the vet is called very quickly he may be able to save the foal's life by intensive antibiotic treatment, but foals that survive are usually backward and do not develop properly.

The most common infection before the introduction of antibiotics was joint ill, caused by certain hemolytic streptococci which cause blood poisoning followed by infection of one or more joints. The foal runs a fairly high temperature and often becomes very lame in one or more legs. The joints most often affected are the hock, stifle and hip joints on the hind-leg and the knee joint on the fore-leg. The joints become very swollen and tender and sometimes fistulae appear between the joints and the skin. This ailment tends to become chronic; the foal develops slowly and loses weight, and if it recovers the damage done to joints and ligaments is often so serious that the animal is never capable of normal work in adulthood. Nowa-

41

days if treatment with suitable antibiotics begins in time there is a good chance of curing these foals. *Always take a new-born foal's temperature at the first sign of infection.* The normal temperature in the rectum of a new-born foal is 37.3–38.3°C, of a mature horse about 38°C.

PNEUMONIA

Occasionally foals 1–2 months old contract a form of pneumonia, usually fairly slow to develop, caused by *Corynebacterium equi.*

Characteristic of this disease is powerful, pumping abdominal breathing; the sounds (râles) associated with pneumonia can be heard over the area of the whole lung. The temperature rises by 0.1–0.2°C every 24 hours. Out of doors the foal seems tired and apathetic, and often lags behind the mare and walks with a laboured staggering gait with the head and neck drooping towards the ground. Abscesses develop in the lung, varying somewhat in size, and with a thick, whitish wall filled with creamy evil-smelling pus. When the temperature rises to about 40°C the crisis is reached, the foal exhibits all the symptoms of blood poisoning and dies within 24 hours. If treated in time, before too many abscesses have developed in the lung, a foal with this type of pneumonia may sometimes be saved by intensive antibiotic treatment.

There are many other bacteria and viruses which can attack new-born and young foals; probably no young mammal is as vulnerable as a young horse. *If there is the slightest suspicion that a new-born foal may be ill, always take its temperature and call the vet immediately.*

WEANING

Weaning is often a difficult stage in a foal's development. Until it is 2–3 months old the foal is almost entirely dependent on its mother's milk, but later it has to obtain food from other sources to supply the needs of a body that is now growing rapidly. Grass, hay, oats etc are broken down in the large intestines with the help of various agents, including enzymes and vitamins. Some foals have difficulty producing these enzymes, and often the production of vitamin B_{12} is inadequate. As a result the foal loses weight and sheds its coat later than normal. At this period of its life the foal is seriously exposed to attack by parasites for the first time; the mare starts to produce less milk, and from the beginning of July the quality of the grass begins to deteriorate.

All these factors coincide to hinder the development of many foals at this age. Worming, vitamin supplements preferably administered via the digestive tract, and other special supplements to the diet often help to correct this rather pathetic and long-drawn-out condition.

The foal, it should be stressed, is very much dependent upon the mare, even though it may seem very independent and not interested in her. To take a foal away from its mother is usually a severe shock that causes anxiety, loss of appetite and unpredictable changes of temperament. There are no definite rules to follow when weaning foals, no ideal method, and indeed almost every breeder has his own method.

In principle a foal should be weaned earlier if its mother is a poor milk producer. Some mares go dry very suddenly and their foals quite simply starve, gaining no weight at all during this period.

The best time to wean a foal is when it is 4–6 months old, preferably in late summer when there is still time for the foal to be put out in the sun to graze as soon as it is fully weaned and independent. Foals should be prepared for weaning in good time by being given a special manger that the mare cannot reach, where they can learn to eat increasing amounts of concentrates and mineral and vitamin supplements. Dried milk is a useful food to use at this time; fed in suitable quantities it is a valuable source of energy and proteins which will tide the foal over the critical period after it has been separated from the mare.

DISEASES OF THE GROWING SKELETAL STRUCTURE

In most bones in foals there are growth plates (epiphyses) at the ends close to the joints, and particularly in the legs. These growth plates consist of highly vascular bone and cartilage tissue, and here most lengthwise bone growth takes place.

The most easily noticed growth plates are those at the fetlock joint at the lower end of the cannon bone and at the knee joint on the fore-leg. If the function of the growth plates is disturbed for some reason, the tissues respond by a sudden sharp increase in the amounts of bone and cartilage produced. This is called epiphysitis, sometimes popularly referred to as rickets.

There are several possible causes of epiphysitis. An extra load may be put on one side of the growth plate as the result of a bad leg posture such as toeing in, toeing out or bow legs. This can cause internal bleeding and impede the blood circulation and the growth of new bone, and may result in deposits of bone outside the edges of a growth plate. This can also be caused by a sudden invasion of intestinal parasites, by deficiencies of minerals such as calcium or phosphorus, or by inadequate feeding, such as the mare running dry or the foal's diet being incorrectly balanced.

One particular form of epiphysitis, often seen in foals 2–4 months old, results in a stiff, careful gait with very upright pasterns and signs of epiphysitis beginning at the lower end of the cannon bone. At this age foals are often out day and night, the ground is often very hard and the grass of poor quality, the mare travels long distances in search of fodder, the flies are very troublesome and the foal never gets a chance to rest properly. All these factors can contribute to damage to the bone structure, often complicated by disorders of the flexor and extensor muscles of the legs. The treatment is to give the foal a complete rest in a loose-box for as long as may be necessary. In the loose-box the foal rests except while suckling. Worming is essential; so too are mineral and vitamin supplements containing the A, D and E vitamins. Care should be taken to correct faulty leg postures and hoof angles in all growing horses; worming must be carried out at the correct time and the diet must contain enough minerals and vitamins.

The growth plates or epiphyses calcify in a fixed sequence; the number of blood vessels is reduced, the soft cartilaginous and bony tissues change to harder, less vascular, more compact bone. The growth plates at the fetlock joint calcify at about 1 year old, the knee joints at $1\frac{1}{2}$–2 years and the elbow and shoulder joints at about $2\frac{1}{2}$–3 years.

It is therefore a very bad practice to subject horses to any hard, tiring training or work until they are three years old, as this can damage the growth plates, causing lameness, pain, stiffness and permanent mental and physical damage.

FEEDING

A horse cannot develop properly or become capable of the performance that its owner requires unless it is fed properly. One needs experience, good judgement and powers of observation to feed horses properly, but success is impossible without plentiful supplies of good quality fodder.

The horse's digestive system is designed to convert very fibrous foods; the horse is still primarily a herbivore. The diet should therefore consist mainly of grass, hay, concentrates and straw. (Concentrates is used here to mean all types of fodder with a high nutritional value in relation to their bulk, and will mainly consist of oats, barley, etc.) Horses also need some more succulent fodder; salt; water; and often additional minerals and vitamins. When making up the ration, think about the horse's needs and the composition of the various kinds of fodder.

A horse needs energy to carry out the normal bodily functions and to be able to work. Energy is given mainly by carbohydrates, to a lesser extent by fats and proteins. Energy requirements vary according to temperament, size and the amount of work the horse is doing. Excess energy is stored as body fat. Most types of fodder contain energy, but hay, the mainstay of the ration, contains relatively little energy in relation to its volume. To increase the energy in the diet, feed concentrates; oats, the most widely used fodder in this class, contain up to 78 per cent carbohydrates, mostly as starch. Barley may be fed in quantities of up to 40 per cent of the total ration of concentrates.

Protein is very important for the development of bone, muscle and other tissues. Pregnant or suckling mares and young growing horses obviously need a lot of protein; so do horses in training or racing. Well made hay, harvested early in the year, is a good source of the proteins, and oats is an important source especially in countries where haymaking is difficult. The body-building constituents of proteins are called amino acids, some of which are present in insufficient quantity in oats. Soya meal and bran should be fed with oats to make up this deficiency.

Horses also need sugar to maintain the health of the intestinal bacterial flora. Hay contains sugar, but molasses, sugar-beet pulp and carrots are richer in sugar and are valuable supplements to the diet.

Fibre in hay and straw plays an important

It is important to feed horses a mineral supplement

44

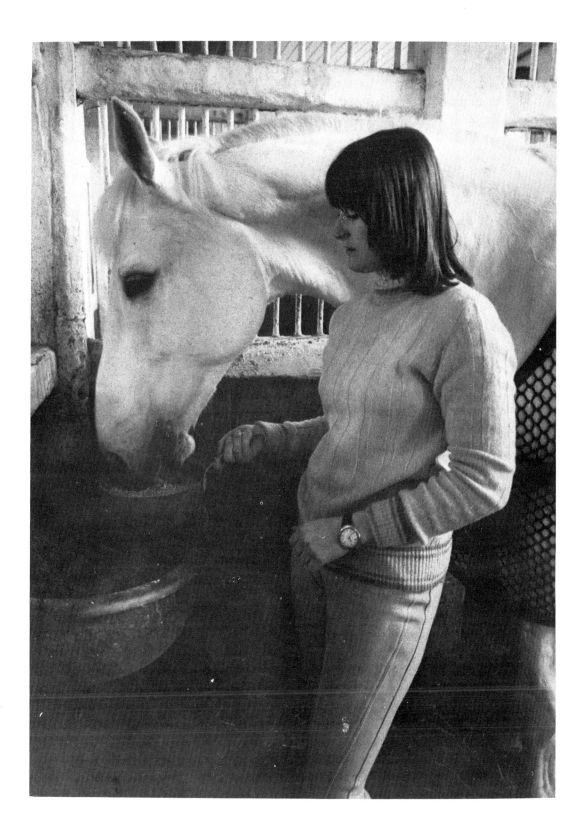

part in the proper working of the intestines; it also satisfies the appetite by adding bulk to the ration, and helps the intestinal flora to function. Disorders of the intestinal flora (bacteria which help digestion) often occur when a horse that has been fed on hay throughout the winter is suddenly put out to grass. Ponies in particular often suffer from digestive disorders in the spring, often leading to acute laminitis. It is wise to ease the changeover from hay to grass by feeding hay for a while after the horses go out to grass.

Suckling mares or horses doing hard or heavy work should not be given so much fibrous fodder. Instead, increase the ration of concentrates in order to give them more proteins and energy. Adult horses doing little or no work can be allowed larger quantities of fibrous fodder.

Mineral supplements. A normal ration usually needs to be supplemented by minerals if the horse is to get enough calcium and phosphorus. Pregnant and suckling mares and immature horses need these minerals most. The main types of fodder may vary in quality, and symptoms of mineral deficiency may then appear unless mineral supplements are given. Foals and young horses may hold the pasterns in a very upright posture and develop swellings around the growth plates particularly at the fetlock and knee joints, and frequently mineral deficiencies in young horses can lead to conditions such as ring-bone and bone spavin. The relative proportions of calcium and phosphorus in the diet are important; recent findings suggest that the diet should contain 1.2–1.4 parts of calcium to 1 part of phosphorus, or 12–14g of calcium to every 10g of phosphorus.

The total mineral requirement will vary with age and also, in mares, according to pregnancy or suckling. It is possible to work out how much of each mineral is present in the various foodstuffs and supplement them with the right amounts of each, but the complexity of the analysis required makes this impractical.

Phosphorus is found in oats and more so in bran. On the other hand, hay contains more calcium than phosphorus. Lucerne and clover hays are particularly high in calcium. Pelleted feeding-stuffs usually carry a label giving an analysis of the contents. One way out of the problem is to supply minerals in a special manger. Horses seem to know which minerals they need; divide the mineral manger into two halves, one for a calcium supplement and one for a combined phosphorus and calcium supplement. Horses also need traces of magnesium, iron, zinc, manganese, copper and cobalt; these are normally included in mineral supplements.

Vitamins. Vitamins are necessary and play a part in various bodily functions. Horses can synthesise certain vitamins such as B, C and D vitamins, but they need vitamins A and E. Vitamin A occurs in carrots, hay and grass, but in winter and spring the amount of vitamin A in stored feeding-stuffs decreases and extra vitamin A is needed. Vitamin D occurs in hay and can be made in the horse's skin during sunlight, but this vitamin also needs to be supplemented during the winter. Vitamin D regulates the absorption of calcium and phosphorus from the gut and its incorporation in the skeletal structure. Vitamin E occurs in bran and oats, but horses doing a lot of work may need extra vitamin E to prevent damage to their muscles.

If the ration is made up from the very best feeding-stuffs, it will usually contain plenty of vitamins, but if additional vitamins are needed there are plenty of vitamin-rich feeds on the market.

46

Salt. Horses need salt in varying amounts according to how much work they do and how much they sweat; a deficiency shows itself as tiredness. Salt licks should be available in the stall and in the paddock or meadow.

The water supply. Horses should have free access to water at a suitable temperature, and it should be good enough to pass for human consumption. If water has to be carried this should be done at least three times a day. A horse will drink up to 50–60 litres per day, but this varies according to the fodder, the amount of work being done, the temperature and the environment. Horses should not be given water for at least an hour after any hard work.

HOW MUCH FOOD?

The amount of food horses need varies greatly. The aim should be to keep them in good condition and capable of doing the work required of them. Pregnant and suckling mares and growing horses have special needs

which should be borne in mind. It is easy to overfeed, and this is often seen in ponies. If ponies are allowed to graze rich leys, particularly in spring when the protein content is high, they can easily get too fat and may possibly develop laminitis. Ponies are often content with a fairly light diet, and are frequently not given enough work.

In discussing the ration it will be assumed that the conventional feeding-stuffs will form the basis of the diet; these are hay, grass, straw, oats, bran, soya, carrots, molasses or sugar-beet pulp, minerals and vitamin supplements. Horse nut concentrates can be fed in place of oats, bran and soya.

Nuts are made of meal, bran, molasses and oil-rich concentrates, with added minerals and vitamins. One of the advantages of nuts is that their composition may be varied by the manufacturers to suit the needs of horses at different stages of life. If oats is replaced by nuts, feed a volume of nuts equivalent to about 75 per cent of the ration of oats.

Horses grazing

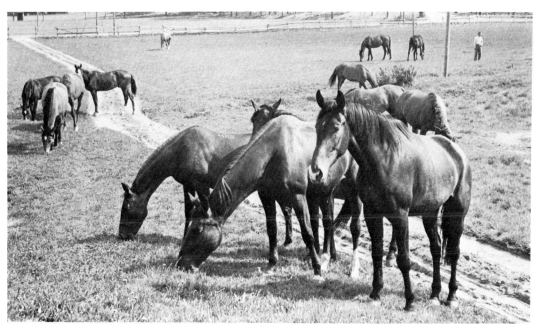

47

Hay should not be fed until November in the same year that it is made. Oats are fed after Christmas of the year in which they have been grown. Boiled barley is fed with great care and is considered to be more suitable for fattening cattle than for feeding horses. There is little feeding value in sugar-beet pulp. It is useful mainly as a bulk food, and again, in spite of prevalent fashion is more suitable for cattle. Carrots or a little molassine meal are a useful additive but need not be fed in every feed.

Grazing. Horses on good grass need no other foods apart from mineral supplements. Keep the mineral trough covered so that it doesn't get wet. When horses are first turned out to grass in the spring they should be given some hay to help the intestinal flora to adapt slowly to the change. Concentrates should be given if the grazing is of poorer quality, particularly when the grazing begins to deteriorate later in the summer. Thoroughbreds tend to lose condition when out to grass, and mares with foals also sometimes need additional concentrates. It should be observed that in some western countries, during the hot summer months, it is customary to bring horses in during the day so that they are not pestered by flies and to turn them out at night.

Pregnant mares. During the autumn and winter and until foaling a mare's ration should be roughly 6–7kg of hay, 2–3kg of oats, 1kg of bran and 3–4kg of carrots each day. Substitute 200g of molasses if carrots are not available. Freely available mineral supplements and any vitamins given as instructed should be included in the ration.

Suckling mares. When lactation begins after the birth of the foal the mare's ration of oats should be increased to 5–6kg. As well as bran it is usual to feed 1kg of soya meal or oil-cake. As a rule the foal will start to eat hay and oats a month or two after birth, and an extra kilo of each should then be added. It is a common fault to overfeed mares in summer, which can also affect foals, which may mean that the skeleton cannot grow fast enough to keep up with their development; such foals may develop very upright pasterns and cocked ankles.

The first year. Foals grow as much in the first year as in the next 3–4 years put together, so their rations must be made up very carefully. Above all they need plenty of minerals and proteins. Well made, early clover hay is an ideal fodder for young horses.

5kg of hay, 2kg of oats and 3kg each of bran and soya meal is a suitable ration. If nuts are used instead, the total ration should be equivalent to about 75 per cent of the conventional fodder. Carrots and molasses should be given to supply the need for more succulent fodder, and mineral and vitamin supplements to complete the diet.

The second and third years. During these years the amount of hay and oats should be increased as the horse's needs increase. The soya meal can be left out.

Racehorses. Horses racing or in training have even larger protein requirements. Increase the amount of concentrates to 6–7kg and include soya meal and bran in the ration. Horses that are worked hard are given more concentrates and less of the bulkier fibrous foods, but the amount of fibrous fodder should never fall below 1kg of hay per day for every 100kg body weight, or the horse's health will suffer. Remember too that the skeletal structure is constantly undergoing renewal, and make sure that the mineral intake is adequate.

Ponies. A pony can get by quite well on hay, straw, minerals and some succulent fodder. If oats or bran are fed only small quantities should be given, except in the case of suckling mares which should be given a suitable ration of concentrates. It is very easy to overfeed ponies, which should be put out in summer to graze on fairly light pastures.

Feeding methods and timing. Horses have small stomachs and should therefore be fed three times a day. Make sure that no food is left in the manger between feeds. If a horse is rested for a day or more the ration of concentrates should be cut by half; on a race day less hay is fed, and no oats for several hours before a race. After strenuous work or exercise a horse should not be fed for at least half an hour.

Fodder quality and hygiene. Horses often suffer from digestive disorders, from conditions similar to asthma, and they can even abort, as the result of being given poor-quality fodder.

Hay should be made early and made well. It should be green and smell fresh, and be free of dust. Be careful to store it somewhere dry.

Oats should have good full grains with thin husks, and should smell pleasant. The grains should be dry and should not stick together in lumps. Examine each new consignment of oats. When feeding newly harvested oats, mix them with oats from the year before, to prevent digestive disorders.

Barley. Treat barley as for oats (above).

Carrots should be fresh and clean. Watch out for rotten carrots.

Sugar-beet pulp should be soaked in water before being fed; if fed dry it can cause blockages in the gullet. Beet-pulp should be soaked the same day as it is fed, because it is liable to start fermenting.

Bedding straw should be of good quality and well dried. Reject any rotten or mouldy straw.

Minerals should be given in quantities that are cleaned up and not left in the manger. If a horse will not eat mineral supplements, mix them with the concentrates. A suitable quantity of minerals would be 50–100g of a combined mineral supplement. Instructions given by the makers should be carefully followed.

CARE OF THE HOOVES

A horse's working life can often be considerably shortened if its feet are not looked after properly, and neglect is a common cause of lameness. Horse-breeders should begin to trim foals' feet when they are 3–4 weeks old, and should trim them regularly every six weeks until they are fully grown, taking any action that may be necessary to correct faulty or mis-shapen hooves. It is also very important to shoe horses as soon as their work makes this necessary, and to have them re-shod every 5–8 weeks, according to the speed at which the hooves grow. The longer a horse can be left un-shod the better; three-year-olds often only need shoes on their fore-feet. Ponies should be shod according to the work required of them. If not shod, watch for sore feet.

WHAT DOES A NORMAL HOOF LOOK LIKE?

The wall of the hoof should be twice as long at the toe as it is at the heels. The height should be the same on each side of the hoof, and the heels should be at equal distances from the ground. The surface of the hoof wall should be smooth and even, and should slope at roughly the same angle on each side. The bottom of the wall should be even and hard, and the sole firm and somewhat arched.

The frog should be well developed, and the bar should turn in towards the middle of the frog.

THE ANTI-CONCUSSION MECHANISM OF THE FOOT

The shock-absorbing tissues in the hooves must be working perfectly if they are to withstand the pressures created when, for example, a trotting horse is supported by only two feet, or when a galloping horse puts all its weight on one foot. These shock-absorbing tissues are the elastic cushion, the plantar cushion, which lies below the navicular bone, and the frog, the sole and the horny wall of the hoof. When weight is transmitted from the body through the long and short pastern bones to the navicular bone and the coffin or pedal bone, the elastic tissues spread outwards under the pressure, which is then transmitted downwards to the frog, which in turn is supported by the ground. The weight also pushes the wall of the hoof outwards, the heels moving sideways 5–10mm, and the heels and the sole sink slightly. These movements within the hoof protect the inner parts of the foot from damage, and also affect the blood circulation within the hoof, their pumping action alternately sucking and pressing on the blood-

Correcting faulty hoof-angles. The shaded parts should be trimmed away. (From Ende, *Die Stallapotheke,* Zurich 1971)

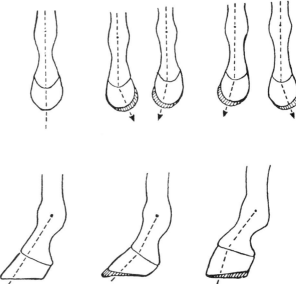

Foal with overgrown hooves

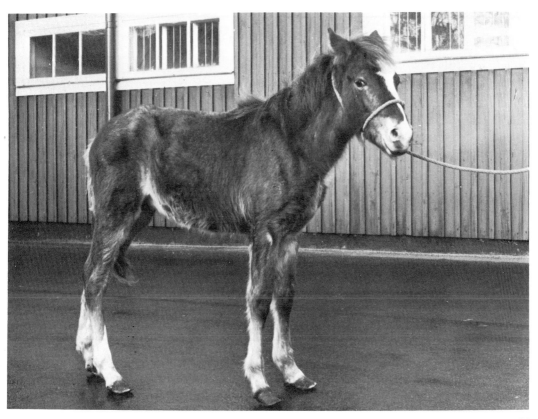

vessels. If the flexibility is impaired, therefore, so is the metabolism of the foot.

The anti-concussion mechanisms function well in horses with normal hooves without shoes. Shoeing always reduces the flexibility of the foot to some extent, so it is important that horses are shod as expertly as possible. The hooves should be looked after properly while the horse is growing, and *regularly* throughout the horse's life. Go to an experienced farrier, and give his work the respect it deserves.

TRIMMING THE HOOVES OF FOALS AND YOUNG HORSES

The hooves should be trimmed first when the foal is 3–4 weeks old. Look to see where the hoof has worn most. The wall of the hoof will be more vertical on the side that has worn most and will slope more gently on the side that has worn least. The less worn side should be pared down until both sides are the same height and the sole of the foot is level. If trimming cannot correct the fault, it will be necessary to fit a half or three-quarter shoe under the worn part of the hoof. If the horse is splay-footed, the inner wall of the hoof will be worn most, or even the toe. Remember that the outside of the toe can also be trimmed back. If the horse is pigeon-toed the position will be reversed. If the horse is shod, the heel of the shoe should be widened on the side which wears fastest.

If the horse has any tendency to knuckle over, the heels should be trimmed accordingly or, better still, a tip shoe should be fitted after the heels have been trimmed.

When dressing hooves, remember that the frog must always be properly supported by the ground.

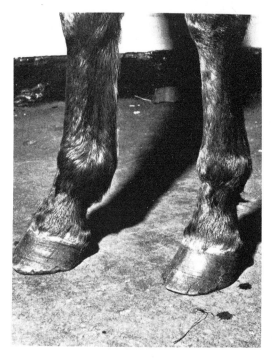

Fore-feet before trimming

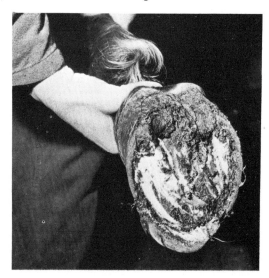

Sole of overgrown hoof

52

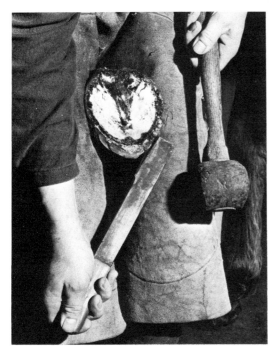

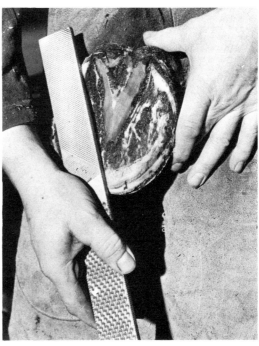

Trimming with a toeing knife and rubber mallet

After trimming the hoof is smoothed off with a rasp

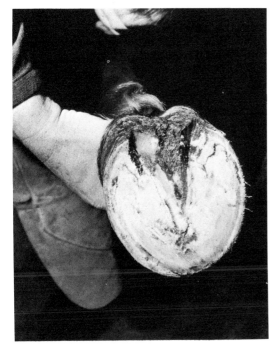

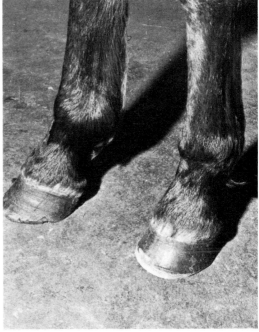

Both pictures above show newly trimmed hooves

SHOEING

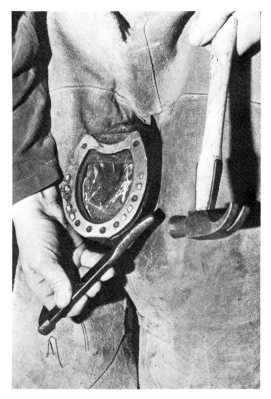

1. Taking the old shoe off. Cutting the clenches

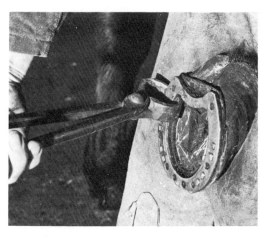

2. Removing the shoe, starting at the heels

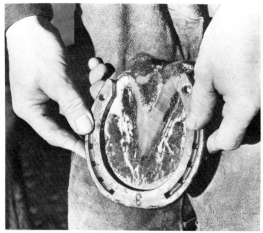

3. Fitting a new shoe

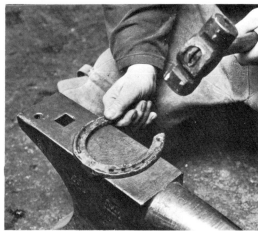

4. Adjusting the shoe to fit the foot

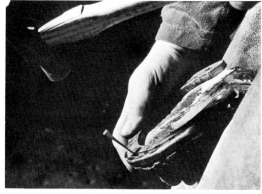

5. The shoe is nailed on

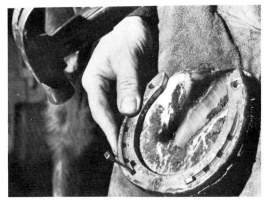

6. Always start at the toe

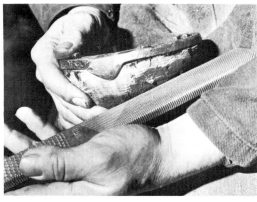

9. Rasping off the burr below each nail

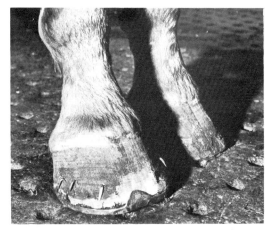

7. All the nails are driven home

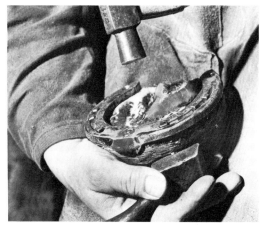

10. Clenching the nails

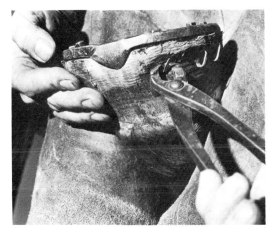

8. The ends of the nails are cut off

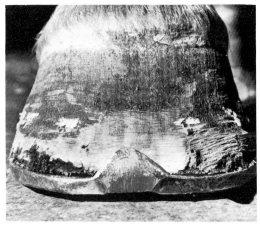

11. Shoeing completed

SURGICAL SHOEING

A lame horse often needs surgical shoes. As well as the shoes for correcting faults already mentioned, there are various types of shoes used to treat various ailments.

When a horse has been treated for an abscess in the foot, entailing the removal of

A. Shoe with sole-plate and set-screws

B. Three-quarter shoe

C. Tip shoe

D. Half shoe

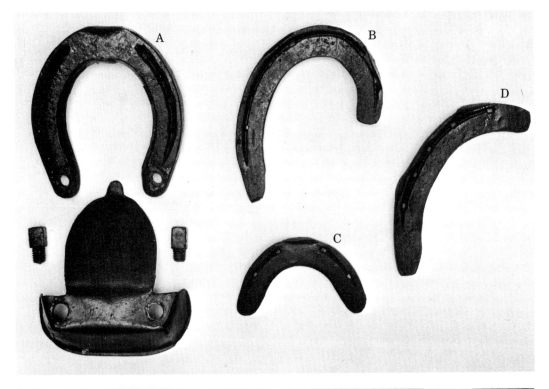

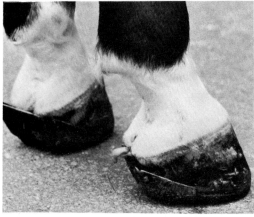
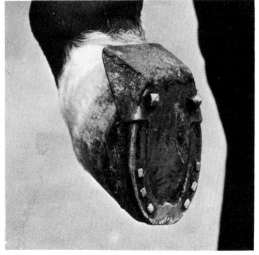

A special shoe with a removable sole-plate used instead of a bandage for treating thrush

56

a small part of the horny sole, the sensitive sole must be protected until the horn has grown again, which is done by fitting a leather pad. This is also done if a horse has thin soles. When treating a horse after a nail puncture, a sheet-metal sole-plate is fastened to the shoe by means of set-screws, so that it can be easily removed each time the wound is dressed.

There are also several types of shoe fitted with rubber pads or, more recently, plastic pads or cushions, which are used to treat conditions such as laminitis, pedal arthritis, pedal ostitis and sidebone.

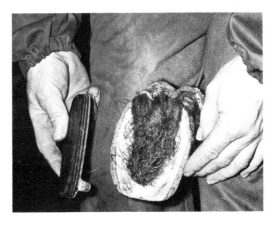

The hoof is trimmed; note the shortened toe. Tarred tow is packed around the frog before the special shoe is fitted

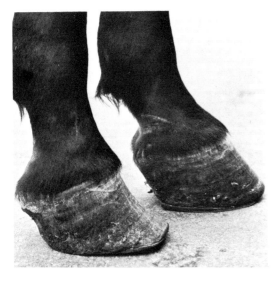

Chronic laminitis with dropped sole on the right fore-leg. Note the concave wall of the hoof

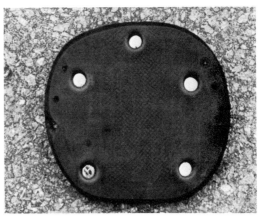

A surgical shoe with a rubber sole rivetted to an iron plate

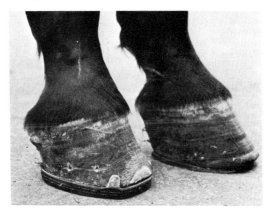

Surgical shoe in place

PARASITES OF THE HORSE

A parasite is a plant or an animal which lives in or on another plant or animal and which damages the host as a result of its own activities and its method of reproduction. Most animals have parasites, and they are a serious problem in domesticated animals.

Parasites are a growing problem in the case of horses. Until about 1945 most horses in Sweden were bred on small farms where the farming rotations (ploughing, cereal growing) reduced the risk of infestations by parasites. Large specialised breeding units or studs were rarer, and the density of horses on pastures was generally so low as to almost eliminate the risk of infection.

Nowadays horse-breeding is concentrated in large stud farms, often running horses in pastures at too high densities. It is too expensive to cleanse pastures by ploughing them up. In general, where large numbers of horses collect either for breeding or riding, at stud farms, riding schools or racecourses, there is always a serious and constant parasite problem.

Parasites can be classified in various ways, for example (a) *by appearance:* roundworms, flatworms etc, (b) *by occurrence:* internal parasites occurring in the stomach, gut, lung etc; external parasites which live on the skin, eg lice and botfly eggs.

The commonest horse parasites are white-worms (*Ascaris*), redworms (*Strongylus*), botfly larvae (*Gasterophilus*) and seatworms (*Oxyuris*).

Lice and botfly eggs and larvae are frequently found in or on the skin.

INTESTINAL PARASITES

Ascaris (whiteworm) is the most typical parasite of foals and young horses. The adults, which live in the small intestine, are large, round worms rather like earthworms, about 25–35cm long. They reproduce themselves by means of thick-walled eggs which pass out in the dung. About a week later a larva develops inside each egg.

The egg's casing is uneven and spiky, and it sticks to fodder and bedding. It is swallowed in fodder or water and returns to the gut where the larva hatches out. The larva cannot develop into a sexually mature adult until it has completed a series of migrations through the body of its host; it burrows through the wall of the gut and is carried in the bloodstream to the liver and then on to the heart and the lungs. Here it leaves the bloodstream, travelling through the lung tissues to the air passages, where it causes irritation and is coughed up and swallowed, thus returning to the gut, where it can develop into a sexually mature adult. During the summer it is quite common to see foals 2–4 months old with a slight brownish discharge from one or both nostrils, accompanied by an obstinate dry cough. These are the symptoms of a serious infestation of whiteworms. The life cycle of *Ascaris* from egg to mature adult takes 2–2½ months.

Ascaris causes serious damage in the small intestine, particularly in foals, disrupting the resorbtion of minerals, vitamins and other nutrients. A foal infested with whiteworms is generally thin and does not do well, with a dull, straggly coat which it fails to shed at the normal time. The abdomen is often very swollen. The disruption of mineral resorbtion can lead to skeletal damage such as epiphysitis at the fetlock joints, and the migrating larvae may spread infection, causing various respiratory infections.

The botfly and its larvae. The botfly (*Gastero-*

philus) is represented in Britain by three species. It is a yellow, brown and black bee-like fly up to 18mm long which lays its eggs on the skin, mainly in places where the horse is likely to bite or lick itself, eg on the forelegs near the knee and on the trunk especially around the shoulders.

On warm still days in July–September the flies attack, and the horses become worried and irritable, often bunching together in flocks with their heads together in an attempt to escape the flies. The female botfly has a long ovipositor under her body. She flies close to a horse's head and rapidly sprays eggs through her ovipositor onto the horse's hair, where they stick on. The eggs are pale yellow in colour, 1–2mm long. After 2–10 days a very active larva comes out of each egg,

Taken during an operation to relieve an intestinal blockage caused by *Ascaris*. The parasites can be seen through the wall of the intestines

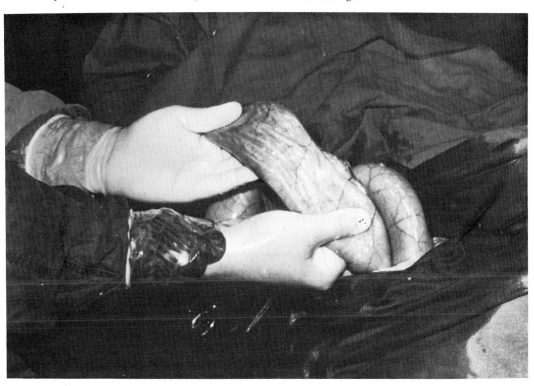

which irritates the horse and makes the skin itch. The horse licks and bites itself, and so the larva enters the mouth. It tunnels into the mucous membrane and migrates via the throat and the wall of the gullet to the stomach, where it bores into and attaches itself to the upper part of the stomach. This migration takes about a month, so the first larvae can usually be found in the stomach around 1 October. The larvae stay in the stomach for 8–10 months and grow to about 20mm long; when fully developed they lose their attachment to the stomach wall and allow themselves to be carried away passively with the contents of the gut until they fall with the dung onto the ground. The larvae change into pupae in the dung, and after 2–3 weeks the casing of the pupa splits and a fully sexually mature botfly emerges, ready to mate and to produce eggs.

Botfly larvae can cause a variety of complaints. While migrating in the walls of the mouth, throat and gullet they can cause local infections, and in the stomach their bites can cause localised inflammation which can disrupt the function of the stomach. Sometimes they have even been known to cause ruptures of the stomach wall. The disruption of the stomach's function leads to digestive disorders and loss of condition.

Redworms (*Strongylus and Trichonema*) are without doubt the most common intestinal parasites found in horses. There are many species of redworm. As adults they live in large numbers in the horse's large intestine, where they attach themselves by biting or sucking to the mucous membrane from which they draw their nourishment. Their life cycles are very complex and vary from species to species; all of them lay thin-shelled eggs which come out in the dung in the stable or in the paddock. The eggs hatch, freeing larvae, which are very mobile and easily climb up the sides of stalls, or up damp grass, and return in the fodder, water or grass to the horse's gut.

The larvae of *Trichonema* enter the walls of the large intestine where they pass through various stages of development before returning fully developed to the large intestine. They are less than 1mm long and cannot be seen by the naked eye.

The larvae of *Strongylus* have very complex life-cycles which differ from species to species. The commonest and most dangerous (*Strongylus vulgaris*) has a larva which bores its way into a blood vessel (artery) and migrates towards the spot where the aorta branches into smaller vessels supplying the various intestines. Here the larvae attach themselves to the walls of the blood vessels and after developing there for a while they return to the large intestine and develop into sexually mature adults. Other migrations through the liver, lungs etc are a possibility. They take 6–7 months to develop, a relatively long time, and when fully grown they are often visible to the naked eye, 10–50mm long and greyish-red in colour.

There is little doubt that redworms cause more damage to horses than any other parasite. In the large intestine the adult redworms suck blood from the walls, and heavy infestation can cause loss of weight and anaemia. More serious is the damage done by the migrating larvae, settling in arteries such as the anterior mesenteric at the base of the aorta supplying the intestines. Here they can cause inflammation (arteritis) which in turn can lead to the blood clotting and sticking to the lining of the blood vessel, often blocking large and small blood vessels and affecting the circulation to parts of the intestines. Clinically this manifests itself as a serious and prolonged attack of colic.

It is probable that the larvae can carry infections from the gut with them on their migrations, causing otherwise inexplicable infections in other organs.

In the large intestine these parasites produce toxins (poisonous waste products) which can affect the whole body. One of the commonest reactions is found in the inner membranes of the joints and of the sheaths surrounding tendons, which react by producing extra synovial fluid. This is seen clinically as an increased fullness in all the joints and tendon sheaths.

Seatworms (*Oxyuris*) are a common intestinal parasite in the horse. They live in the large intestine and the rectum. The females are larger than the males, up to 100mm long, though their size is fairly variable; they are grey-white in colour.

When the horse is standing quietly in a stall or loose-box the mature female seat-worms crawl out through the anus and lay their eggs there. Their movements on the skin cause itching and irritation; the horse rubs itself to ease the itching, and the eggs fall to the ground. The eggs re-enter the gut on fodder, straw and grass, hatch out, and the adults develop in the large intestine, reaching sexual maturity at around 5 months old.

When the horse tries to ease the irritation around the anus caused by the female worms crawling there, by rubbing itself against a projection in the stall or the paddock, it often causes sores and inflammation around and on the root of the tail. The hair in the tail is damaged and tangled up, the horse becomes restless and kicks bars and walls, and this can lead to sores and lymphangitis in the hind legs.

Foal suffering from infestation by lice

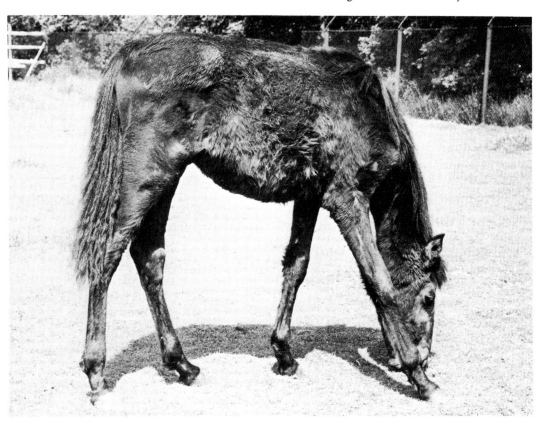

61

EXTERNAL PARASITES

Lice. This parasite lives on the skin particularly on the throat and the sides of the neck and, in a heavy infestation, over the whole body. The movements of the lice, and their bites, cause inflammation, which causes irritation which the horse attempts to relieve by rubbing itself against fences and branches. Large patches of skin can become completely bald and a secondary skin inflammation may develop. In a serious case a young horse may lose weight and suffer from anaemia.

Lice spend their entire life-cycle on the horse's skin. They lay eggs which stick to the hair near the surface of the skin, hatching after 5–10 days. An adult louse is 2–3mm long, yellowish brown in colour. Infestations only occur in winter and early spring, as the lice cannot develop except at low temperatures and in the horse's winter coat.

Lice are transferred from one host to another mainly by direct contact, but they can be passed on in brushes and saddlery. Very few lice survive the higher summer temperatures, but in the cooler autumn temperatures a new generation can soon develop.

Treatment is to clip long-haired horses (burning all the hair cut off!) and to treat the skin with a suitable powder or liquid. Treatment should be repeated after 10 days, and all stalls and loose-boxes should be cleaned carefully and treated so as to kill any lice that have fallen to the ground.

DIAGNOSIS OF INFESTATION BY PARASITES

Diagnosis of parasite infestation is usually by means of an examination of the dung to determine how many eggs it contains. This examination will reveal if parasites are present and if so which sort; though a negative result should be treated with reservation, since this may mean simply that the actual droppings examined contained no eggs. There may be large quantities of eggs in the next droppings.

Note that the presence of botfly larvae (*Gasterophilus*) cannot be revealed through examining the dung since the eggs are laid on the horse's skin.

CONTROL AND TREATMENT OF INTESTINAL PARASITES

Prevention. Prevention is the most important of the measures that can be taken against parasites. Daily mucking-out of stalls and loose-boxes is essential. Whenever possible the dung should be composted or ploughed under arable ground; it should never be spread on places where horses graze.

Cleaning should be done with high-pressure equipment when possible. Mangers and other fodder containers should be planned so that contamination cannot occur, and it is also important to ventilate stables well, as a warm, damp environment speeds up the parasites' development to the larval stage.

Hygiene in the pasture is often neglected. Damp, low-lying ground liable to flooding encourages parasites. Watering places should be dry and as high as possible; if possible water should be laid on to a suitable trough that can easily be cleaned. Pastures should be split into smaller units so that horses can have frequent changes of pasture. A very good method is to plough up pastures and grow cereals on them for a year or so before sowing grass again, but this is an expensive method and not always practicable. It is advisable to graze a new grass ley first with cattle or to take a hay crop; newly sown grass-land should be reserved for mares with foals. Harrowing with light harrows now and then breaks up the droppings and spreads them about, which hinders the development of parasite larvae, exposing them to the sun and drying them out.

Veterinary treatment. Worming with chemical preparations is the only method of any importance at present for ridding horses of intestinal parasites. A great deal of research is being done all over the world to develop biological treatments (vaccines) but up to now with little success.

A good worming preparation should comply with several criteria: it should be harmless to the host animal, cheap, and not liable to the risk that the parasite may get used to it (develop resistance). It should also taste pleasant, so that the animals will willingly eat it, and it should be effective, killing a very high proportion of all species of horse parasites. Worming should always be supervised by a vet, who should prescribe a suitable preparation and the correct dosage.

Horses in the peak of condition in training for a race should *not* be wormed too soon before the race. Choose a break between races, and plan a course of treatment during longer periods of rest or breaks in training.

All worming should be done to a schedule planned beforehand. Worming once, eg in the autumn, is quite inadequate. A single worming simply puts the problem forward for a while without achieving any solution. Treatment of intestinal parasites is always a constant battle between the parasites and the horse-owner. Be consistent; worm at the right time with the most effective preparations; follow a proper schedule; and consult your vet.

SUGGESTED WORMING PROGRAMME

YOUNG HORSES

Jan	Feb	Mar	April	May	June	July	Aug	Sept	Oct	Nov	Dec
1			**2**		**3**			**4**			**5**

Redworms (*Strongylus and Trichonema*) **Ascaris**	Worming in the middle of the grazing period is recommended	**Redworms** (*Strongylus and Trichonema*) **Ascaris** **Botfly**

Worm at least twice during the spring months. As soon as young horses are taken in for the winter it is very important to worm for the four parasites named above.

ADULT HORSES

Jan	Feb	Mar	April	May	June	July	Aug	Sept	Oct	Nov	Dec
	1			**2**		**3**			**4**		**5**

Redworms (*Strongylus and Trichonema*) **Ascaris**	**Redworms** (*Strongylus and Trichonema*) **Ascaris**	**Redworms** (*Strongylus and Trichonema*) **Ascaris** **Botfly**

Check for parasites by dung analysis. Do not worm a horse in top racing condition; always worm when the horse is not racing.

BROOD MARES

Jan	Feb	Mar	April	May	June	July	Aug	Sept	Oct	Nov	Dec
1			**2**		**3**			**4**			**5**

Jan	Feb	Mar	April	May	June	July	Aug	Sept	Oct	Nov	Dec
Redworms (*Strongylus and Trichonema*) **Ascaris**				**Redworms** (*Strongylus and Trichonema*) **Ascaris**				**Redworms** (*Strongylus and Trichonema*) **Ascaris** **Botfly**			

Worm a mare before she foals, but not in the last month before she is due. Further wormings should be done before going out to grass and while out to grass. When mares are taken in for the winter the two wormings shown above for the four parasites named are important.

FOALS

Jan	Feb	Mar	April	May	June	July	Aug	Sept	Oct	Nov	Dec
								4			**5**

Jan	Feb	Mar	April	May	June	July	Aug	Sept	Oct	Nov	Dec
Ascaris *1st worming at 1.5–2 months	**Ascaris** *Trichonema* *2nd worming 4–6 weeks later			Foals should also be wormed while out to grass				**Redworms** (*Strongylus and Trichonema*) **Ascaris** **Botfly**			

*Timing of 1st and 2nd wormings applies to late-born foals too; ie worm according to the foal's age and not according to the time the horses are put out to grass.

INFECTIOUS DISEASES

VIRUS DISEASES

Influenza in the horse is caused by a virus very similar to that which causes influenza in man. There are two known types, called A1 and A2. There are occasional outbreaks of influenza in unvaccinated horses.

Incubation takes from 2 to 3 days.

The symptoms are, first of all, fever lasting about 24 hours. The horse becomes lethargic and has a watery nasal discharge. The musculature becomes tender and the horse moves very stiffly. After a day or two a persistent hacking cough develops. If the horse is rested and no complications develop, recovery takes between 1 and 3 weeks. If the horse is exposed to any form of stress, eg work, cold or bad weather, bacterial secondary infections may develop, causing a new fever, and the nasal discharge will turn yellowish.

Treatment in cases with no complications consists of rest for at least 2–3 weeks. It is important to check the temperature daily. If secondary infections develop these must be treated with antibiotics or sulpha drugs until completely cured. It is very important to keep the stable clean when influenza is present.

Prevention. The best method is to vaccinate, which can be done when a foal is more than a month old. A good level of immunity is not developed until two weeks after the second vaccination, which is done 6–12 weeks after the first. Horses should be re-vaccinated once a year. Vaccination carries no risks even at the later stages of pregnancy, but should be avoided if a horse is racing or in training; if such horses are nevertheless vaccinated, they should be rested for 14 days. The risk of complications after vaccination is very small. Research in the UK has shown that these occur in 0.63 per cent of cases, where an abscess develops at the site of the injection. The corresponding figure for Sweden is about 0.8 per cent. Several investigations have demonstrated the efficacy of vaccination. Immunity lasts for about a year; the commercially available vaccines are double vaccines which give immunity from both types of influenza.

An infected stable should be isolated for at least 14 days after the last horse's temperature returns to normal. The influenza virus is very infectious; the rate of infection is usually 70–90 per cent, and infection can be from horse to horse or via humans or equipment.

Equine herpesvirus, often referred to as virus abortion, is a common virus disease, causing inflammation of the upper respiratory tract in young horses, known as 'runny nose'. In older horses which have had the disease several times the symptoms may pass undetected, except in pregnant mares, where it causes abortion. The disease is most common in autumn and winter, young horses often going down with 'runny nose' when they are brought in for the winter.

The incubation period for runny nose is 2–10 days.

The symptoms in young horses are a temperature of 39–40°C for about a week, with loss of condition and appetite during that time. Sometimes swellings appear on the legs and the abdomen; sometimes diarrhoea; but the symptoms can often be extremely mild. Recovery takes 1–2 weeks without any special treatment. Secondary infections producing a purulent inflammation of the upper respiratory tract may also develop.

Pregnant mares which are infected abort after from 3 weeks to 3 months. The foetus is infected and is aborted particularly between the 8th and the 11th months of pregnancy. If the mare is infected at a very late stage of pregnancy the foal may be born living but generally does not survive. Usually the mare can conceive again without difficulty after an abortion. The disease is very infectious; all the horses in the stable will normally catch it unless there is some immunity already. Abortion varies in frequency, but can occur in as many as 90 per cent of infected pregnant mares.

Immunity is short-lived; horses can be infected again after 3–6 months, although immunity against abortion generally lasts for as long as two years.

Preventive measures are very important. Horses that are racing should never be housed in the same stable as pregnant mares. When a new mare comes to a stud-farm she should be kept in quarantine for three weeks before being allowed to come into contact with the other horses. There are effective vaccines against virus abortion. Vaccinations should be repeated annually or whenever the horses are liable to become infected, eg when there is an outbreak in the district.

Infectious equine anaemia (swamp fever) is a virus disease of horses which first shows itself as a fever up to 40–41°C lasting 3–5 days. The horse's general condition is seriously affected, and it may suffer from oedema (abnormal accumulation of fluid outside cells) under the chest and abdomen and in the legs. Sometimes horses develop jaundice and in acute cases may even die. More usually horses appear to recover after the first fever, but suffer another attack of fever 3–4 weeks later, a pattern that can be repeated for a long time, during which the horse will gradually deteriorate, losing weight and becoming increasingly anaemic. The disease can last for several years but the horse never recovers. Formerly it was a common disease in cold-blooded horses in the north of Sweden; it was eradicated in the 1950s but recently there have been occurrences of the disease on and off in southern and central Sweden.

This disease is contagious, passed on from one horse to another, but it can also be passed on via equipment and instruments. The virus may be present in blood, urine and saliva.

The only way to control the disease is to destroy the animals affected. The disease has caused considerable losses in the USA and France.

Equine viral arteritis occurs in America and in western Europe and derives its name from the way the virus attacks small blood vessels (arterioles).

Incubation takes 2–10 days.

The symptoms begin with fever up to 41°C. The eyes water and the nose discharges more mucus than usual, and the mucous membranes of the eye become inflamed and swollen, which is why the disease is sometimes called 'pink eye'. Oedematous swellings appear on abdomen and legs, and sometimes there is diarrhoea. The horse recovers after about 2 weeks, if there are no secondary infections, but pregnant mares invariably abort.

The treatment is rest for 3–4 weeks, and special treatment to restore the condition of any animals that have been particularly badly affected. There is no vaccine for this disease, and strict isolation is the only way to combat it.

Equine encephalomyelitis is a dreaded disease among horses on both American continents. There are three main strains, Eastern Equine Encephalomyelitis (EEE); Western Equine Encephalomyelitis (WEE); and Venezuelan Equine Encephalomyelitis (VEE). The virus is spread by insects, which spread the infection to mammals and birds. A serious outbreak of VEE occurred in Central America in 1970, where hundreds of horses were affected and many died. Even human beings were infected. This led to widespread measures being taken against the disease, and strict isolation being enforced. 2.8 million horses were vaccinated in 19 states around Texas, and measures to eradicate insects affected an area of 5.2 million hectares.

All types of equine encephalomyelitis cause a high fever and symptoms from the central nervous system. Death occurs in about 90 per cent of cases. There is no cure, but horses can be protected by vaccination.

This disease does not occur in Europe. There are strict quarantine regulations for all horses originating in USA, which also need certificates and blood tests to show that they are free of the disease. Any exporting country is banned from importing horses to Europe if an epidemic occurs there and until the epidemic has died down.

African horse sickness is a very infectious, rapidly developing virus disease with a very high death-rate. As the name suggests, it is mainly an African disease, but there have been outbreaks in Asia and even in Spain. The virus is spread by insects.

BACTERIAL DISEASES

Strangles is caused by the bacterium *Streptococcus equi*. It is an acute infectious disease, which not infrequently follows on after a virus infection. The disease occurs throughout the world and in Sweden it occurs in most parts of the country. Its occurrence has become more frequent as the result of increasing importation of horses.

Infection takes place either as a result of direct contact or contact with infected mangers, fodder, equipment or even via human beings.

Incubation takes 4–8 days.

The symptoms begin with fever and loss of appetite, the temperature rising to 40–41°C. Other symptoms are a nasal discharge and a cough. A few days later swellings develop in the lymph glands around the throat and behind the lower jaw. In some of the lymph glands abscesses develop, bursting when ripe and discharging pus. Some abscesses do not burst and must be opened surgically.

Treatment. Apart from the surgical treatment mentioned above, a horse with strangles should be given a course of penicillin injections over a period of at least a week, after which the horse should recover from the infection. It should be allowed to rest for at least a month, and should be given an ECG test before being allowed to resume training, as it has been shown that inflammation of the heart muscle often accompanies a case of strangles.

Complications. If a horse is not treated it may develop bastard strangles, caused by the infection spreading to lymph glands in the chest and abdomen. Even joints may be affected. The chances of recovery from bastard strangles are slimmer, particularly in young horses or horses in poor condition, which can develop a very severe and sometimes fatal form of the disease.

Other complications are roaring, whistling and anaemia. Occasionally anasarca (see p 142) follows strangles. Symptoms are pronounced swellings on the head and neck, trunk and legs. The disease is difficult to treat and is sometimes fatal.

Isolation should be strictly enforced for at least 14 days after an outbreak of strangles. This period should be extended if new cases occur; we have known cases where the outbreak has gone on for six weeks. There is no vaccine, but serum will give protection for about 14 days.

A horse that has had strangles is immune to the disease for the rest of its life.

Glanders is a contagious disease caused by the bacterium *Loefflerella mallei*, which attacks the nose, lungs and skin. The disease is usually fatal in both the chronic and the acute forms, and can spread to human beings.

Glanders is a disease that thrived most in wartime, and was first described around 300 BC. It is a notifiable disease in the UK.

WOUNDS

The horse's environment and the uses to which it is put often expose it to the risk of cuts and wounds, particularly in spring and summer. Barbed wire is an all too common cause of deep and complicated wounds; its use in fences should be forbidden. Badly designed stables with sharp projections can cause punctured and lacerated wounds; dark, badly designed cow-byres are all too often used as stables, especially around large towns.

Road accidents involving horses are a more common occurrence nowadays, when horse transporters leave the road or stray horses run onto roads; accidents of this sort can cause extensive incised or contused wounds. Wounds are classified according to how they are inflicted as incised, lacerated,

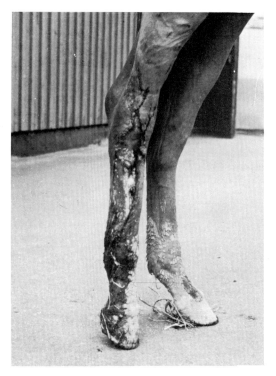

Cut on hind-leg caused by barbed wire

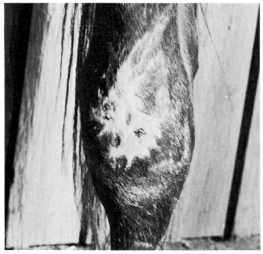

Barbed-wire cut on the hock after plastic surgery

punctured and contused wounds, and are also described as open and closed wounds. In the latter case the soft parts under the skin are damaged but the skin is not broken.

Horse-owners and grooms ought to be able to form an opinion about the position and extent of a wound, but most wounds will need the attention of the vet. Nonetheless, first-aid is very important, and an antiseptic solution should be used.

TYPES OF WOUND

Incised wounds are characterised by smooth, profusely bleeding surfaces and clean-cut edges. Such wounds are caused by the horse walking through or on glass or being cut by other sharp objects. Such wounds heal best if stitched as soon as possible after the injury happens. While waiting for this to be done the owner should examine the cut, wash the area around it and apply a proper bandage or, if the bleeding is very profuse, a compress. In the case of arterial bleeding, which can be recognised by the pulsation and by the bright red colour of the blood, it may be necessary to apply a tourniquet as well as a compress. This is possible with a leg wound. Rubber tubing makes a good tourniquet. Don't leave it in place for more than an hour. Wounds which are stitched usually heal within 12–14 days, but full strength is only reached after about a month. Until then the horse should be rested.

Lacerated wounds are generally flap-like. They can be caused by barbed wire, nails and other projections, and are commonest on horses' legs. Often there is a pocket

Chronic lymphangitis (big leg)

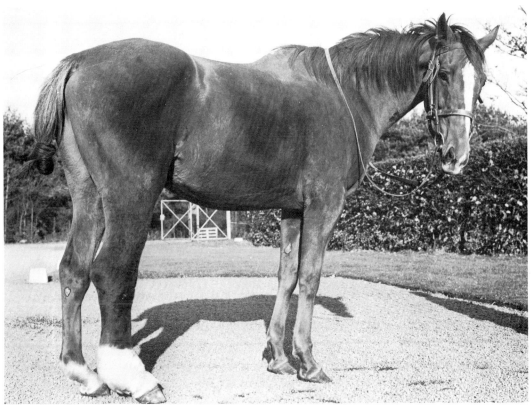

deeper than the opening of the cut, where dirt and the wound's secretions can collect. This pocket should be kept open and allowed to drain freely until the wound no longer discharges.

Punctured wounds have only a small opening in relation to their depth. They bleed very little or not at all and can easily go undetected. A punctured wound is often infected and may affect joints, tendon sheaths and the bone's covering membrane (periosteum). For this reason punctured wounds are particularly serious and should be seen by the vet as soon as possible. If an infection develops the symptoms are a locally raised temperature, swelling, raised body temperature, increased sensitivity to touch and lameness if the wound is on the leg (lymphangitis). Lymphangitis is very liable to recur and develop into what is known as elephantiasis or big leg.

Punctured wounds can harbour the bacilli that cause tetanus (lockjaw), and a dose of tetanus antitoxin or toxin is indicated. The disease is described more fully below. When sharp objects penetrate the hoof causing punctured wounds they nearly always cause a hoof abscess. The owner should notice where the object, a nail for example, was lying in the hoof before being removed, as this will help the vet to assess the damage. A nail can sometimes penetrate the pedal joint or the navicular bursa, in which case medical treatment may take 6–8 weeks and the horse may be lame for up to half a year.

Contused wounds are caused by horses kicking each other, falling, hitting bars while jumping etc. Common sites are the knees, the elbows, the points of the hocks, the points of the hips and around the eye sockets. These injuries are also seen in horses after a bad attack of colic. The skin is often lacerated and dirty. The wound cannot be stitched but must be allowed to heal naturally, which often takes a long time. The wound must be dressed carefully every day, and it will usually fall to the owner to attend to this.

HEALING

Healing processes. Before the wound begins to heal a natural cleansing process removes the damaged tissue and attacks the bacteria in the wound. In a wound with no complications this takes 24–48 hours, but in contused or large, lacerated wounds it can take several weeks. The vet can speed up the process by cutting out damaged or infected tissue. The would then heals by rebuilding blood vessels and connective tissue from the edges of the wound. The space between the sides of the wound fills with granulation tissue, which is very rich in blood vessels. It lacks nerves and is therefore insensitive. When the gap is filled with granulation tissue, which protects the wound from infection, the skin grows across from the sides.

Healing by 'first intention' is a term reserved for healing when the wound is stitched or when the edges of the wound are close together without being stitched. Healing takes 12–14 days.

Healing by 'second intention' takes place when stitches burst or when a wound is large and lacks skin. Healing can take several months, and plastic surgery is often necessary. This is a method of transferring normal skin in small pieces from the back of the thigh to the granulation tissue, where they are 'grafted on' and form islands from which the skin re-grows. Skin transplants are often necessary in the case of wounds on the anterior surface of the hock or the lower parts of the legs.

Healing depends on several factors. Healthy young animals heal better than older ones, and animals that eat and drink little after an operation do not heal so well. The position of the wound can be very critical; wounds on the eyelids or lips, which have a good blood-supply, heal faster than wounds on the legs, where there are fewer blood-vessels. Infections delay healing.

COMPLICATIONS

All accidental wounds will contain bacteria that can cause infections. The animal's inherited natural resistance, the type of wound, its position, the amount of contamination and the way the wound is treated are the factors which will determine whether an infection develops. Insignificant punctured wounds reaching tendon sheaths or joints can cause highly dangerous infections.

A typical infected wound will be swollen, painful and will cause fever and the development of pus. Sometimes lymphangitis will also occur (inflamed lymphatic vessels), and sometimes this will develop into general blood poisoning. Sometimes an infected wound bursts after having been sewn.

Modern antibiotics and sulpha drugs give us good prospects of curing most infections. If a course of these drugs is begun it should not be broken off too soon. Often a test is necessary to determine which antibiotic or sulpha drug should be used (ie one to which the bacteria are not resistant).

SOME SPECIFIC WOUND INFECTIONS

Tetanus is a horrific disease which usually develops as a consequence of a punctured wound, often in the hoof. The bacterium which causes tetanus (lockjaw) is widespread in the soil and also lives in the horse's gut. It also has a dormant form (spores) which is extremely resistant and therefore has a very good chance of survival. If spores enter the

Wound with severe skin loss

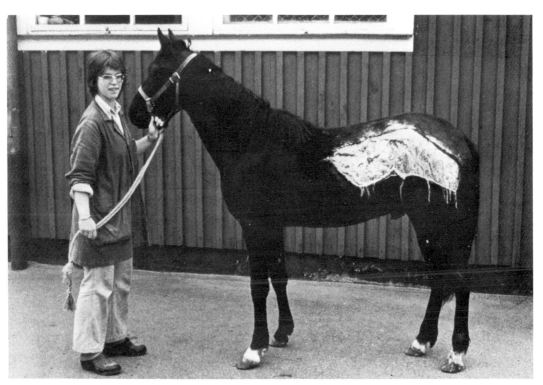

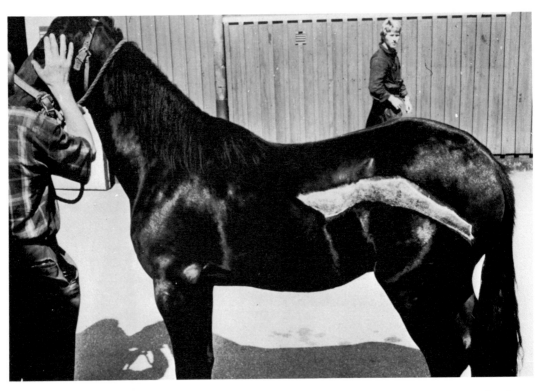

Healing three months later

body through a wound the dormant stage ends and the bacteria multiply, producing a poison (toxin) which damages nerve tissue.

Incubation, ie the time between infection and the appearance of the disease, can take anything from 4–5 days to as long as 3–4 weeks. In new-born foals the incubation period is very short.

Symptoms. The first symptom that the horse's owner notices is that the horse becomes very stiff in its movements. The horse then starts to have difficulty moving its jaws. An early symptom is spasm of the third eyelid, which becomes more obvious if the horse's head is quickly lifted up. Soon the horse takes up the characteristic 'sawing horse' stance, with the tail slightly lifted and the ears erect. In serious cases it will become unable to chew

or to swallow, and will find it difficult to stand, which is why it is usual to support it with slings to stop it falling over. It is important that the horse be kept quiet and in the dark, but in spite of intensive care, including artificial feeding and injections of both sedatives and substances to relieve the muscle spasms, it is unlikely that the horse will recover. At least 50 per cent of affected horses either die or have to be destroyed. Horses which retain the ability to chew and swallow and which can be kept on their feet usually survive, but recovery takes at least four weeks.

Prevention. This dreaded and, for the horse, extremely painful disease can be prevented, and every horse-owner ought to be obliged to vaccinate his horses against tetanus. The Swedish Veterinary Institute recommends:

1. First injection at 1 month old

74

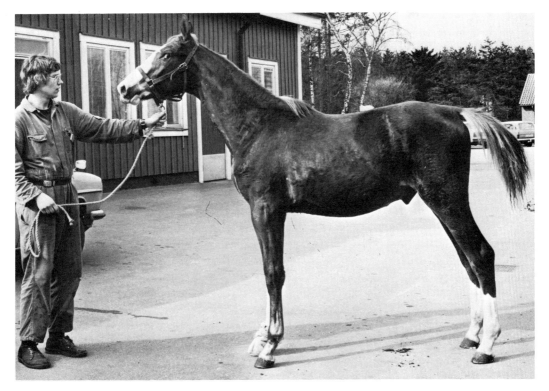

Lockjaw

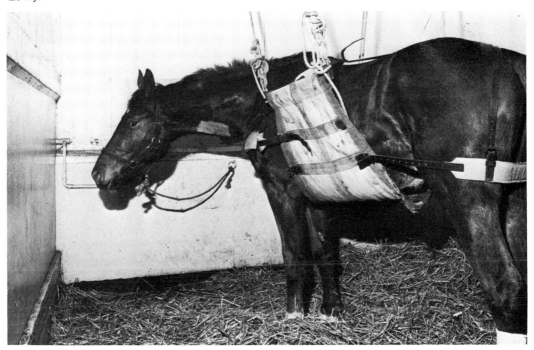

Horse with lockjaw supported in a sling

2. Second injection six weeks later
3. Third injection a year later

This course of injections should protect the horse for ten years, but re-vaccination is nevertheless recommended every time the horse is wounded.

The new-born foal should be protected by vaccinating the mare during the last two months of pregnancy. Antibodies are then transferred to the foal, which is thus protected for the first month.

Wounded horses that have not been vaccinated are given antitetanic serum, which gives protection by means of antibodies for about 14 days. It is usual to inject vaccine and serum at the same time.

Botriomycosis is an infection associated with wounds, caused by a bacterium (*Botriomyces equi*), which gives rise to tumour-like swellings which contain small abscesses and fistulae.

Botriomycosis occurs in the skin, the lymph glands and the udders. In some cases the infection can attack bone tissues, and is then extremely difficult to cure. The infection can begin in small, insignificant wounds and spread through the body via lymph and blood vessels. It sometimes arises as a complication following castration.

The causal organism is responsive to penicillin but treatment takes a long time. Botriomycosis is, however, rare nowadays.

Gas gangrene is an unusual infection that occurs as a result of extensive and serious tissue damage. It is caused by bacteria which produce gas. The period of incubation is

Botriomycosis

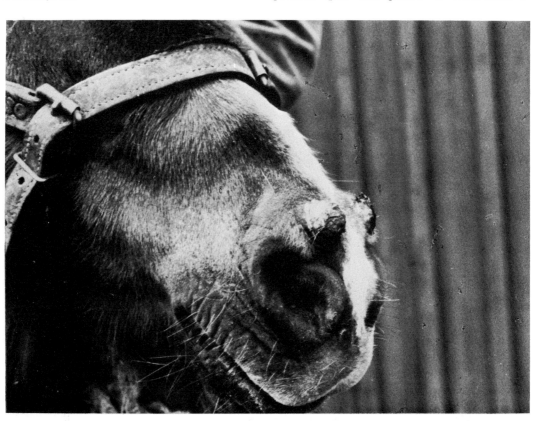

short, 24–48 hours. Symptoms are hard swellings, painful on pressure, with gas collecting in the tissues. The horse becomes weak and lethargic, runs a high temperature, loses its appetite and moves with difficulty. Death often occurs within a day or so.

Proud flesh is a complication that follows wounds, and refers to the cauliflower-like granulations that grow out from wide, open wounds where the skin has been lost. It is often seen on the anterior surface of the hock and on the lower parts of the legs if the membrane (periosteum) covering the bone is damaged. Proud flesh must be reduced to the same level as the surrounding skin for healing to take place, so it must be cut away with a knife or burnt off by a caustic astringent from time to time. Skin grafts are often necessary, as mentioned above.

COMMON WOUNDS IN SPECIFIC SITES

Head wounds. The head is rich in blood vessels, which makes healing easier. Wounds to the eyelids and lips should be stitched if 'cosmetic' considerations are important.

Eye wounds. These are usually caused by flying glass or sharp projecting objects. Eye damage should always be treated as soon as possible, as even an injury to the surface of the cornea can leave a permanent mark. The best way of bandaging a horse's eye is to lift up the third eyelid and temporarily fasten it so as to cover the eyeball. Cuts on the cornea are very painful and the horse becomes photophobic; for this reason the horse should be put into as dark a stall as possible and not allowed out in daylight.

Mouth wounds are caused by sharp teeth and by teeth at unsuitable angles etc. It is important to examine the mouth regularly. If the cause is removed the injury will heal.

Saddle galls are becoming more common, partly because of carelessness. When a horse is ridden the skin is under pressure, sometimes sideways pressure, and small breaks in the skin caused by this pressure can be infected by bacteria. These 'sitfasts' are very difficult to treat, and often the horse has to be rested for several weeks, not being ridden until the infection has been cured. Preventive measures are important; the horse's saddle cloth should be cleaned regularly, and both saddle and saddle cloth should fit properly; if any infection is present the back should be cleaned with an antiseptic every day.

Pastern wounds often have similar causes to saddle galls. Small cuts and abrasions are easily caused by earth or sand getting behind bandages, boots etc. This can, if allowed to become infected, cause inflammation of the pasterns (grease or mud fever). This should be treated at least twice a day, before and after work, by cleaning with an antiseptic such as iodine and a protective antiseptic cream. In serious cases of grease it may be often necessary to give general treatment with sulpha drugs or antibiotics to prevent inflammation of the lymph glands (lymphangitis). An effective method is to combine a chloromycetin spray with silver nitrate ointment alternated with vitamin A and D ointment.

Impalement is when a branch or a stake enters the body, frequently at the groin or behind the shoulder-blade. Sometimes the object can penetrate to the abdominal or chest cavities and cause fatal damage. If only skin and muscle are damaged, healing is usually satisfactory provided the object can be removed. Sometimes several operations have to be performed before the whole or parts of the object can be removed.

PARTICULARLY COMPLICATED WOUNDS

Wounded tendons. Wounded tendons are commonest at the pastern joint, where both the deep and the superficial flexor tendons may be affected, causing lameness. After operating the leg should be put in plaster. Healing can take a long time, sometimes as long as a year, and there is a risk that the horse will become chronically lame. Young horses have a better chance of complete recovery. Severed extensor tendons heal much more quickly, and the chances of their function being unimpaired are always good.

Wounded tendon sheaths. Wounded tendon sheaths always cause severe lameness, and infection sets in within a few days. These injuries must receive prompt treatment. The tendon sheath must be syringed clean and treated with an antibiotic, and then sewn up. Healing is relatively slow, from 3–4 weeks to several months if a fistula develops.

Impalement

Wounded joints. Wounds in the joints are, if that is possible, even more serious than wounds to the tendon sheaths. Treatment is hospitalisation with a long course of antibiotic treatment sometimes lasting for 3–4 weeks. The horse must rest in a loose-box until the lameness disappears. Wounded joints are very painful and painkillers should be given at the acute stage, as in other painful conditions.

Wounded bones and bone membranes often go unnoticed by the owner and the horse is rarely treated until several weeks after receiving the injury. They occur mostly on the pasterns and cannons, where the bone tissue is very close beneath the skin. Such wounds often lead to infections in the bone together with exostosis (bony growth on surface of bone). Healing takes a long time; sometimes an operation may be necessary to remove dead bone tissue. A long course of antibiotic treatment is always necessary.

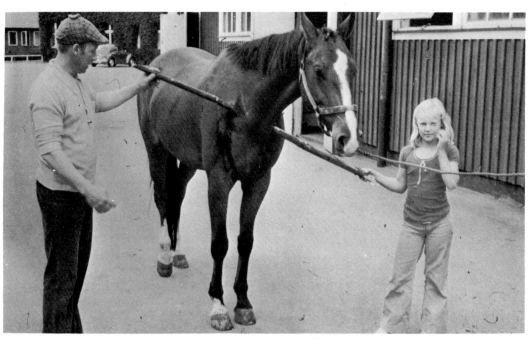

Closed wounds are wounds below the surface of the skin caused by blows or kicks, when the surface of the skin is not broken. A bag-like swelling forms, containing blood and lymph. Such wounds are treated with soothing, cooling ointments for a day or so and then with ointments which speed up the resorbtion of the contents. If the swelling has not been reduced noticeably after 14 days the contents can be drained and substances injected to promote quicker healing. The horse should be rested to lessen the risk of bleeding starting again.

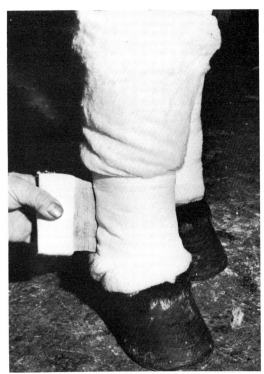

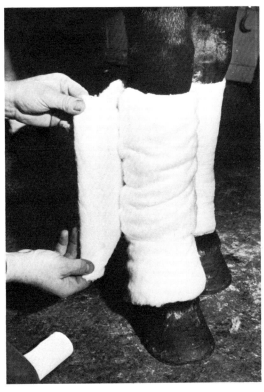

Left and opposite
Bandaging pastern and cannon. Always work upwards

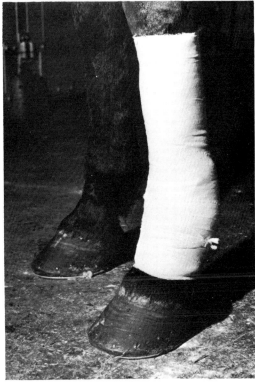

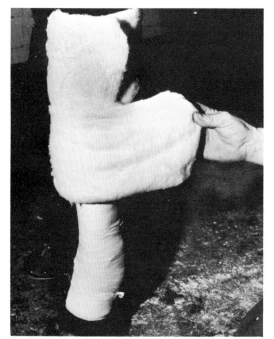
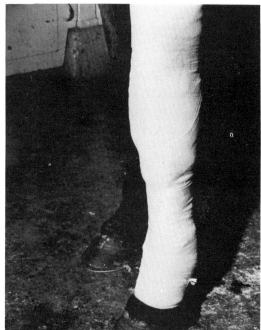

Knee bandage. Note the careful padding

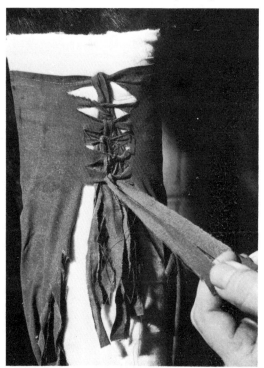
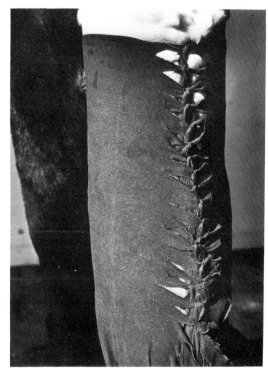

An outer linen bandage is put on to hold the bandage in place

80

THE MEDICINE CHEST

Every horse-owner should have a medicine chest; its contents should include the following materials for treating wounds:

Antiseptics. Tincture of iodine is widely used and is not harmful to the tissue if used at the right concentration. If strong iodine tinctures are not sufficiently diluted they may cause a reaction in the skin.

Kaolin or Animalintex for use as poultices,

A–D vitamins in fish liver oil or ointment are very good for the treatment of wounds that heal slowly and for hoof care.

Copper sulphate solution is a very useful preparation for treating chronic wounds. It has a low pH and stings when applied. It kills bacteria, encourages the sloughing of dead tissue, but does not damage living tissue. It also helps to coagulate blood to a certain extent.

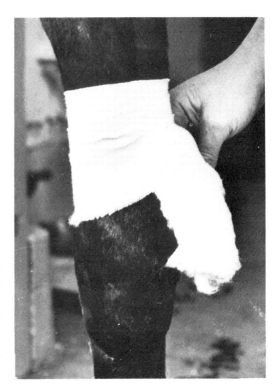

Putting an elastic bandage on a swollen knee. The elastic adhesive bandage should not be stretched

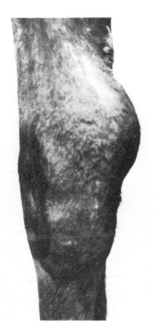

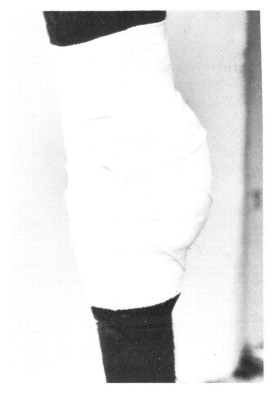

Surgical spirit in a 70 per cent solution is useful for treating abrasions, eg caused by saddlery chafing.

Soap should be available for the preliminary mechanical cleaning of wounds.

Cotton-wool and gauze should be available for bandaging and first-aid.

There are divided opinions as to whether antibiotic ointments and sprays should be kept in medicine chests in the home, as there is a risk that they will be used uncritically and lose their usefulness. They should be supplied by the vet for use in particular cases.

Hock bandage. Careful padding and bandaging are important around the point of the hock

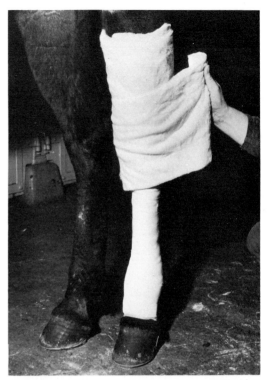

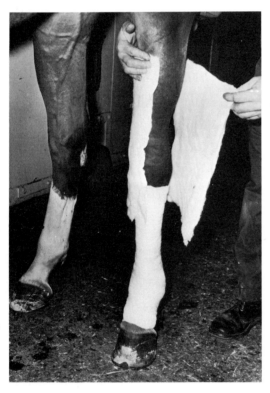

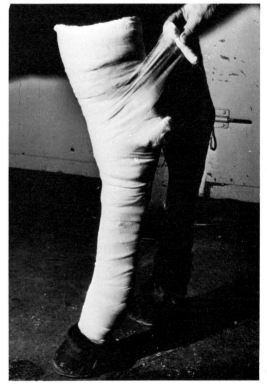

LAMENESS

Lameness is a disturbance of the natural gait caused by the horse trying to reduce pain. This disturbance will be most obvious, according to its severity, either in the horse's walk or when it trots. Acute pain may even be detected when the horse is resting, as it will continually take the weight off the affected extremity or extremities. Lameness can occur in one or more legs simultaneously, as in laminitis, when both fore-legs or all the legs may be affected. In such cases a horse will spend as much time as possible lying down. A general joint- or muscle-inflammation can also cause disturbances in the gait affecting all four legs. Short, stiff and jerky movements are typical of these cases. Even diseases of the central nervous system, the brain and the spinal cord, can cause gait disturbances, often in the form of lack of co-ordination of the leg movements.

Lameness can be the result of either difficulty in supporting the weight or of difficulty in moving the body. The former type generally has its cause in the lower part of the leg, the latter in the upper part. In almost all cases of lameness pain is involved. Riders often talk of a horse being bridle lame. In the opinion of the writers there is no such thing; the explanation lies rather with the rider's bad conscience for riding a lame horse.

Sometimes a horse will show other signs of dissatisfaction when being ridden or driven, by sticking its tongue out when being ridden, for example, or by pulling to one side when being driven at higher speeds. Be sure to examine the teeth in cases of this kind. Sharp edges, often when losing a tooth or teeth, can lacerate the mucous membranes in the cheeks and cause a lot of discomfort.

It has long been customary never to ride or drive a lame horse. In dressage, the most distinguished of all equestrian events, lameness automatically disqualifies. It is to be hoped that this will always remain so.

A lot of people put great faith in strong blisters, which are very widely used to treat lameness. The larger the swelling or the amount of fluid produced, the more faith people seem to have in their efficacy. From a biological point of view this is quite wrong, apart from the unwarrantable suffering caused. Healing can only be delayed by such large, artificial swellings in the tissues. Blisters should be light, often repeated and should preferably not cause any swellings.

DIAGNOSIS OF LAMENESS

When the vet is called to a lame horse he will follow the pattern of the examination chart (overleaf) unless it is obvious that the

83

cause of lameness is, for example, a stone or a nail that has entered the hoof, or if he discovers some other type of wound. The full examination is very comprehensive, but it is necessary in order to be able to make a fairly accurate diagnosis, to begin a suitable course of treatment, and to be able to assess the horse's prospects.

EXAMINATION CHART
Medical history (*anamnesis*)
Pedigree
Performance (records broken, prize money etc)
Age
Races run
Last race
When and how did the horse become lame?
The symptoms of the lameness
The horse's appetite
The horse's fodder
Any previous treatment

Examination
At rest
Condition, general health, conformation, development of the musculature, weight distribution, body temperature etc
In motion
Walking, turning, trotting, between the shafts, ridden
Palpation
General
Detailed
Diagnostic aids
Flexion tests
Diagnostic injections
Nerve blocks
Rectal examination
X-ray examination
Blood tests
Examination of the synovial fluid
Examination of faeces

84

Diagnosis
Treatment
Therapeutic exercises

Medical history. The medical history or *anamnesis* is very important. It is essential to know how long the horse has been lame, how the lameness began, if the horse's appetite has been normal or if it has had a change in its diet, and whether it has had an accident; the owner should be asked about the horse's pedigree, its breeder, and records it may have broken or any races it may have won, together with any details of earlier veterinary treatment.

The horse's ration with its mineral and vitamin content should also be included in its medical history. Many ailments of muscles, joints and tendons are caused by inadequate feeding.

Examination. The horse should be examined first when at rest. The development of the musculature and the horse's general health are assessed. Less well developed muscles in one shoulder or on one side of the croup indicate a disorder high in the leg. Often it may be advisable to take the horse's temperature, as acute laminitis or muscle inflammations can raise the body temperature. The horse's way of standing should also be noted; normally it will take the weight off the leg affected; if two legs are affected it will continually shift its weight to ease first one leg, then the other. The positions and axia of the bones are studied, and note is taken of any large ringbones, splints or windgalls, etc. This general examination of the horse often gives very helpful information; it is not safe to concentrate on any one detail early in the examination.

The horse is next examined in motion, first while *walking,* then *turning* and after that at the *trot*. There is considerable skill in showing a horse correctly, which should be taught to all young helpers, as it is a part of horsemanship well worth preserving. The horse should be bridled and always on the leader's right-hand side. At a walk the end of the reins should be held in the left hand. The horse is always turned to the right. At the trot the leader lengthens the amount of rein given to the horse and holds the end of the reins in the right hand, looking straight ahead and not at the horse.

Study the way the horse puts its feet down on to the ground and how it moves its legs forward. A pronounced double action in any step indicates pain in the horse's toe. The way a horse turns can be interesting; if it puts its hind-legs forward under the body, it has pain in a fore-leg, and vice versa.

The hind-legs should be examined when the horse is moving away from the examiner, and the fore-legs when the horse is moving towards him. Lameness that occurs at a walk or at a trot is categorised on a 1–5 scale. Lameness of class 5 is when the horse does not support any weight at all on the leg in question. An aid to detection is to observe the nodding action of the horse's head; the more it is accentuated the worse the lameness. If the lameness is not detectable when the horse is being led, the horse may be driven or ridden. In the case of thrombosis in the arteries in the hind legs lameness only develops after a period of exercise, though when it does occur the symptoms are very characteristic.

Showing a horse. Contact between the leader and the horse is with the eyes as well as the bridle

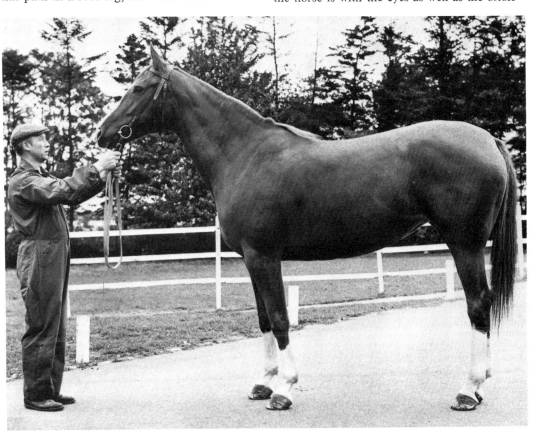

The next stage of the investigation is *palpation*, which means that one feels the various parts of the leg with the hands. Always start by checking whether the horse has a stronger pulse in the common digital arteries in the feet. If this pulse is detectable and if it throbs strongly, suspicion will immediately fall on the hoof. It should be inspected, using hoof testers (pinchers). If the horse is fitted with sole-plates, these should be removed. Many ailments affect the hooves, for example nail perforations, nail binds, inflammation of the sole, hoof abscesses, cracked hooves, treads, pedal ostitis, fracture of the pedal bone etc.

The leg should then be examined, working upwards from the pedal joint to the pasterns and fetlocks, examining also the ligaments and tendons in the pasterns, the deep and superficial flexor tendons, the suspensory ligament, the joints at the knee on the fore-leg, the elbow and shoulder regions. On the hind-leg the procedure is repeated, working

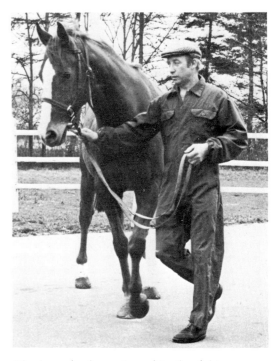

The horse is always turned to the right

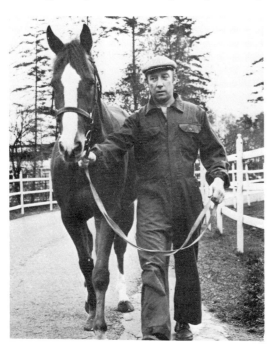

Showing a horse at a walk. Note the way the reins are held

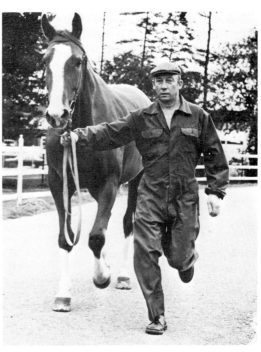

Showing a horse trotting. The reins are now held less close to the horse and the end taken in the right hand. The leader looks straight ahead

86

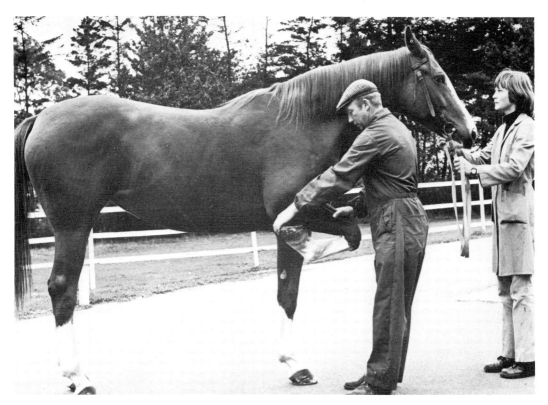

Flexion test on fore-leg

Flexion or bone spavin test on hind-leg

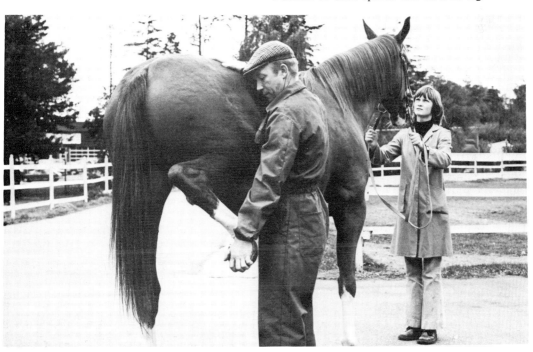

upwards and including the hock, the stifle and the hip joints. The back is also examined, paying particular attention to the development of the muscles and any sensitivity to pressure.

Diagnostic aids. At this stage diagnosis is sometimes possible, but usually further investigation is needed, using what are known as diagnostic aids:

Flexion tests
Nerve blocks
Radiography (X-rays)

Flexion tests can be done on the whole leg or with one joint at a time. If after the test the horse holds the leg up in the flexed position before putting it back on the ground, this will indicate a condition such as bone spavin, and indeed this test is sometimes called a spavin test.

Nerve blocks help to locate the source of the lameness. The nerves of the pastern, fetlock and cannon-bone regions can be anaesthetised, or injections can be made direct into joints or tendon sheaths suspected of causing pain. The most usual joints to which this is done are the fetlock joints on all four legs, both of the upper sections of the knee joint on the fore-legs, the shoulder joints and the various parts of the stifle and hip joints.

Examination per rectum may be extremely useful in the diagnosis of diseases, for example of the blood-vessels of the pelvic and abdominal cavities, which may cause lameness.

Radiography. When the source of the pain has been located, it is usually to take an X-ray; usually it is as well to X-ray the corresponding part of the sound leg for the sake of the comparison, as the normal range of variations is quite wide.

Radiography can reveal a crack, a fracture, a chipped bone, a cyst, etc, but often fails to show the disorder. Diagnosis should never be based wholly on the results of radiography. Clinical observation must be included in the diagnosis.

Blood tests are also an important part of the examination, involving analysing the number of white and red corpuscles, the hemoglobin content, the presence of certain muscle enzymes, calcium, phosphorus and so-called alkaline phosphatase. The latter can give information about the condition of the skeleton.

Examination of the synovial fluid (the lubricating fluid in the joints) can also be useful, as can examination of the faeces, which may show the presence of parasites.

Examination of the teeth is included for reasons mentioned above.

The results of the examination are collated with the information given by the owner or trainer, and the whole used to make the diagnosis and prescribe treatment. In many cases the diagnosis may be uncertain, which will be reflected in both the treatment and in aftercare.

Therapeutic exercises are the last stage of treatment and convalescence. The programme of exercises should be drawn up for the individual horse and the particular injury, and progress must be regularly monitored by the vet.

DISEASES OF THE HOOF

Nail binds and nail pricks can be caused by shoeing. The horse will be sensitive to the hoof testers and the pulse in the leg will throb. The nail should be removed and the hoof bandaged with a compress containing an antiseptic. A hot bran mash poultice is commonly used.

Nail perforations. The horse may often tread on nails without doing any serious damage. But if a nail penetrates the frog it may cause very serious damage in the vital tissues deep within the foot, such as the deep flexor tendon, the navicular bursa and the pedal joint, in which case the vet's help should be sought as soon as possible.

Nail perforations also bring a serious risk of tetanus.

Bruised sole is a common condition which results when a horse with thin soles loses a shoe or when a horse which is normally shod suddenly has to go unshod. Bruised sole usually affects the fore-feet, and treatment consists of cold compresses on the hoof followed by fitting a suitable (surgical) shoe as soon as the worst pain begins to abate.

Corns are characterised by bleeding in the sensitive sole, usually in the angle between the wall and the bar. They are caused by faulty conformation of the foot, incorrect shoeing, riding long distances on hard surfaces etc. A corn can develop into an abscess.

Treatment consists of removing the shoe, trimming the hoof and applying a cold antiseptic compress. A shoe with a leather or sheet-metal sole is fitted later.

Hoof abscesses are common occurrences, often developing very suddenly, with serious lameness, throbbing pulse, sensitivity when the hoof is tapped, a warm hoof and not infrequently a swelling in the leg to above the fetlock. In the early stages it is often difficult to locate the abscess, but if action is not taken the pus, which is often black, will force its way out at the coronary band or at the heels according to the position of the abscess. Hoof abscesses can be caused by nail pricks, nail binds, nail perforations or even cracks in the horny sole. This last is encountered often in young horses spending a lot of time in meadows where the ground is bare and frozen. A hoof abscess should be opened thoroughly, but only by an experienced farrier on the instructions of a veterinary surgeon.

Laminitis is usually a disease of the whole

horse but with its most prominent symptoms occurring in the feet. A horse with laminitis is generally ill, has a fever and sweats. Both fore-hooves, and occasionally all the hooves, become inflamed; the horse finds it difficult both to stand and to walk, and moves with the hind-legs tucked forward under the body, taking jerky, double-action steps. Generally the heels are put down first, and the toes eased down afterwards.

Laminitis can have its origin in the large intestine as the result of incorrect feeding, abrupt changes of fodder etc. It can also occur in connection with an infection of the uterus after birth. Nowadays laminitis caused by over-work is rarely seen. The treatment is to remove the cause. The diet should be rectified and the horse given laxatives to remove the harmful contents of the gut, antihistamines and phenylbutazone, and cold compresses on the feet.

Shetland and Gotland ponies are particularly prone to this illness.

Acute laminitis is often complicated by dropped sole, in which the pedal bone moves round in the hoof, and in extreme cases its point penetrates the sole. Surgical shoes must be fitted, and often refitted four or five times at six-week intervals until the dropped sole is eliminated and the horse fit to work again. Important preventive measures are to change the diet gradually and to be sure that the afterbirth is not retained too long after foaling.

Complete hoof bandage

1. Cotton wool is wrapped round as far as the fetlock joint

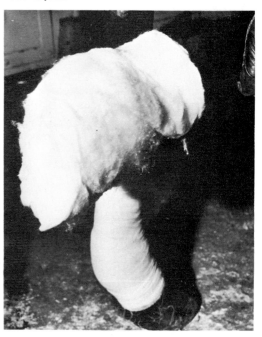

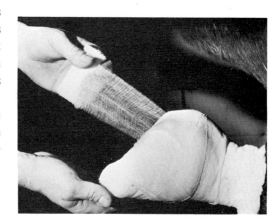

2. The hoof is bandaged with gauze

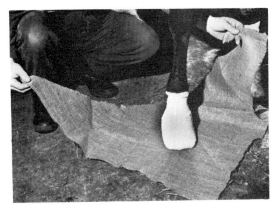

3. A protective hessian bandage is put on as shown here in five stages. The bandaged hoof is first put in the middle of a triangular piece of hessian

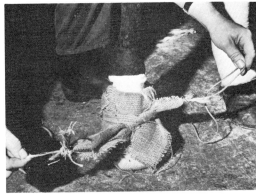

6. String is fastened to the ends of the hessian and taken several times round the bandage to hold it in place securely

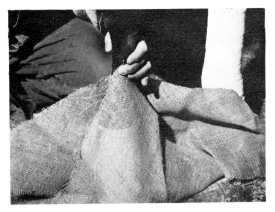

4. The front corner is folded back

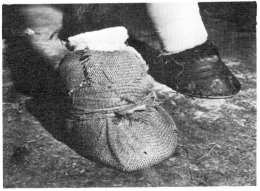

7. The finished hoof bandage. The lower surface should be tarred to make it more durable

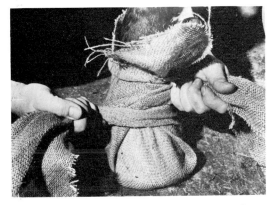

5. The side corners are crossed over on the front of the hoof, taken round the pastern and tied at the front after the front corner has been folded down

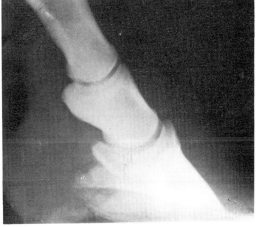

Dropped sole following laminitis

Cracked hooves (sand cracks) are commonest in American trotters, and usually on the insides of the fore-hooves. Cracks can run from the coronet to the bottom of the wall, and can bleed, indicating damage to the soft interior of the hoof.

An effective treatment is to remove the shoes, but this is not always possible. If the crack is bleeding or infected it must be trimmed and the crack filled with plastic. When healing begins the edges of the crack can be held together by rivets to allow the horse to get back to work.

Transverse cracks may be caused by treads; these should also be trimmed and filled with plastic.

Treads are common, and are caused by the horse treading on its own or another horse's foot, especially during the winter when horses are being transported while wearing frost studs or frost nails. Treads can damage the coronary band and loosen the hoof wall. Before transporting horses all such projections should be removed if possible, especially on the insides of the shoes.

The damaged horn should be trimmed away and a compress put on, after which the horse can normally go back to work as usual.

Brittle hooves or hooves with poor-quality horn are often white (unpigmented). The horn cracks and breaks up and the shoes work loose easily, frequently being lost. Often this fault is hereditary, and horses with fragile, brittle hooves should not be used for breeding.

There are certain measures that may be taken to improve the quality of the horn, such as good feeding with plenty of minerals. Experience has also shown that rubbing the coronary bands with fat every day can be very beneficial. The shoes should have toe- and side-clips to stop them coming off.

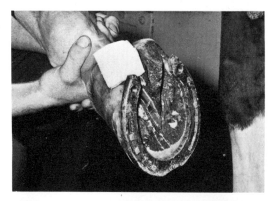

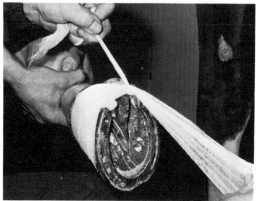

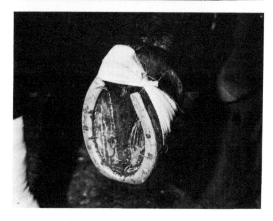

Bandage for treads and other injuries to the coronary band

92

Keratomae are growths of extra horn inside the hoof wall, caused by local inflammation with adhesion of the laminae and an abnormal horn growth as a consequence. This presses on the pedal bone which atrophies, and the pain makes the horse limp. A keratoma must be removed surgically, and the horse will be lame for at least two months after the operation.

Thrush is a degeneration of the frog, often beginning in the central cleft.

Usually several hooves are affected. The cause is lack of attention to the foot and standing in soiled bedding. Treatment is to trim away all rotting and loosened horn and pack tarred tow around the frog.

In severe cases a special shoe with a removable sole-plate is fitted. Thrush can be prevented by keeping the bedding dry and cleaning out the hooves every day.

Sidebone is a condition which, in our present horse population, is not the important cause of lameness that it was in the days of heavy horses, in Sweden mainly of the Ardennes breed. Acute cases of sidebone, often complicated by pedal ostitis and navicular disease, were then common, leading to chronic lameness. Professor Erik Åkerblom, in the early days of the Swedish horse-registration scheme, campaigned vigorously to prevent horses with sidebone, among other conditions, being used for breeding purposes. Sidebone is hereditary.

Horses have two cartilages in each foot which can be felt by palpation above the coronary band on the inside and outside of each foot. This cartilage is normally elastic and, together with the plantar cushion, forms part of the anti-concussion mechanism of the foot. In cases of sidebone the elastic cartilage is changed into hard, bony tissue, and in the Ardennes breed large bony deposits are also formed.

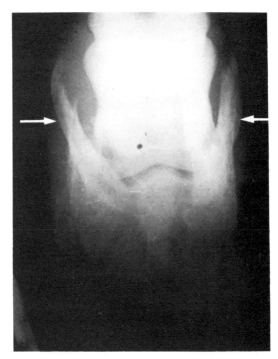

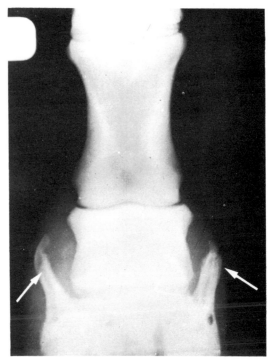

Sidebone

93

Nowadays hardening of the pedal cartilages without any bony deposits is often detected incidentally to the examination of lameness in half-bred horses, usually of the heavy type, and in trotters with French ancestry. These sidebones usually do not cause lameness, but attention is drawn to these cases since mares and stallions with sidebones should not be used for breeding. There are quite naturally cases of sidebones acquired rather than inherited, caused by trauma.

Quittor is an abscess in one of the pedal cartilages accompanied by a purulent discharge, caused usually by an injury, a tread, a puncture wound or by trapping a foot in the bars of a partition in the stable, etc.

The affected horse develops a serious limp and a considerable swelling in the coronary band above the damaged pedal cartilage, with an intermittent discharge of pus. Modern medicaments and surgical treatments usually restore these horses to health within a couple of months. Formerly this condition required major surgery and at least six months' convalescence.

DISEASES OF THE BONES AND JOINTS

Cracks or fissures can occur in every part of the skeleton. The commonest are cracks in the long pastern, the pedal bone, the sesamoid bone and the splint bones. Trotters seem particularly liable to cracks in the long pastern and sesamoid bones.

Cracks in the radius (fore) or the tibia (hind), as the result of kicks or blows to the part of the bone that lies directly below the skin, can be very treacherous. All cracks can lead to complete fractures, which in the case of these two bones would be catastrophic.

Cracked bones typically cause a sudden, severe lameness. In some cases the pain recedes quickly and the lameness may have almost disappeared after a couple of days. If a horse with a cracked bone is put to work before the crack has completely healed, there is a serious danger of a full-scale fracture.

Radiography is the only way to be certain if there is a crack or fissure. Sometimes it is necessary to operate, screwing the sides of the crack together, in order to prevent future disability. (For example, cracks in the long pastern running down towards the pastern joint.) If this is not done there is a risk of ringbone developing and causing chronic lameness. Healing may take anything from two months to half a year. If a crack is diagnosed in the radius or tibia of an adult horse, the animal should be supported by slings for about 2 months, and an operation to screw up the crack may be necessary.

Broken bones can happen to horses of all ages. A new-born foal can be trodden on by its mother, or an old horse can get a complicated fracture while trotting or galloping in a paddock.

The symptoms can vary according to which bone has been damaged and how it has been broken.

Broken neck. If a horse breaks its neck, it will lie motionless on the ground. It loses consciousness and its eyes roll rapidly in their sockets (*nystagmus*); usually it bleeds from one of its ears. This may happen when a hind-leg gets entangled in a halter chain or the horse falls in the loose-box or at a fence.

If the spinal column is broken the horse will either be paralysed completely or in the hind-quarters, depending on which vertebra has been broken. A horse with a broken back cannot be cured and should be put out of its suffering as quickly as possible.

It is important to know that concussion can cause a fallen horse to lie unconscious.

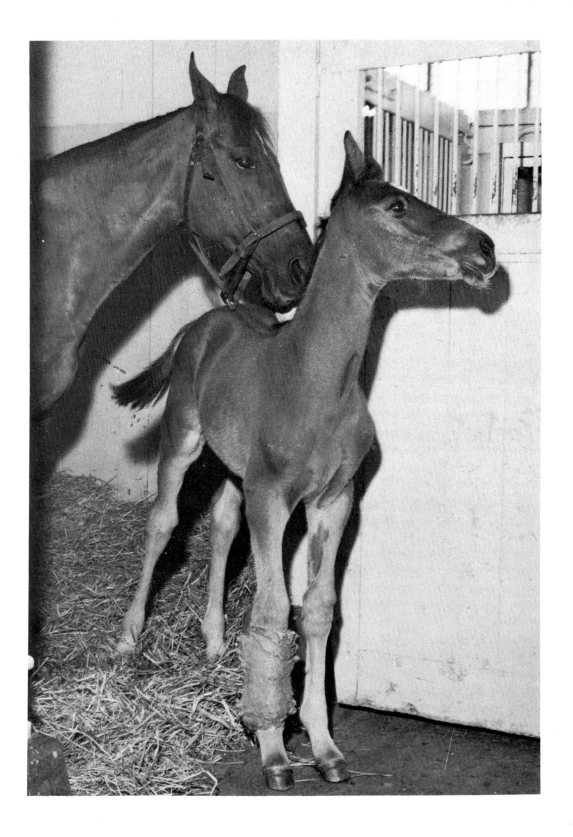

Do not have the horse put down in a panic without giving the vet a chance to see the horse.

A broken pelvis may only affect the ilium or 'wing' of the pelvis, causing a permanent lowering of one side of the croup. The horse may still be capable of work but a horse with this injury will not be suitable for dressage events.

More complicated fractures which damage the actual pelvic girdle can also heal satisfactorily, leaving the horse unimpaired, though fractures involving the hip joint will result in a permanent disability.

Most vets have to form a judgement about fractures of this type by means of a *per rectum* examination. At present only the radiography department at a veterinary clinic has the personnel and the resources to fully investigate such pelvic fractures and give a correct prognosis.

Treatment of pelvic fractures involving the main pelvic girdle is at least two months supported by slings, and complete recovery may take up to six months. Whether to begin treatment or not must be decided on the merits of each individual case.

Complete fractures of the main, long, leg bones such as the humerus, radius, femur and tibia are usually incurable in adult horses of normal size with the techniques at present available. Exceptions are certain fractures at the ends near the joints which can sometimes be operated on with a reasonable hope of success. The prognosis for foals, young horses and ponies with fractures of the main long bones in the legs is often more favourable.

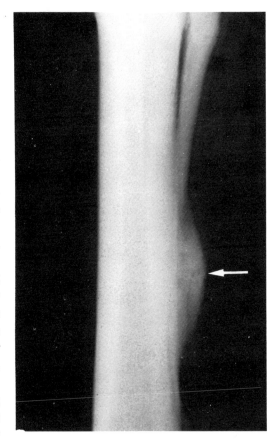

Exostosis

Foal after operation for broken cannon-bone

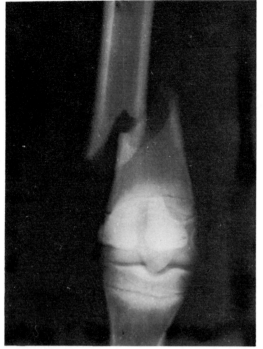

Fractured cannon bone

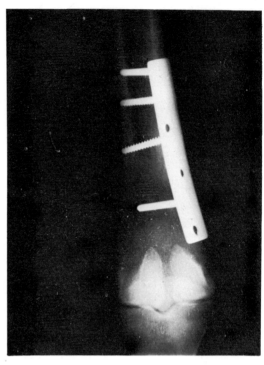

Healing after six months

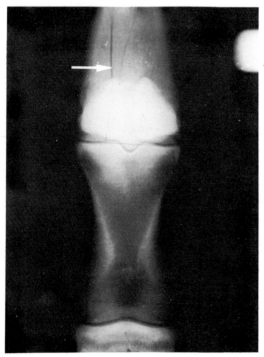

Fracture at lower end of cannon bone

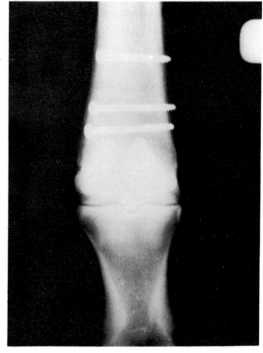

Healing after three months

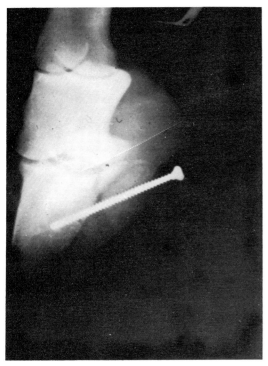

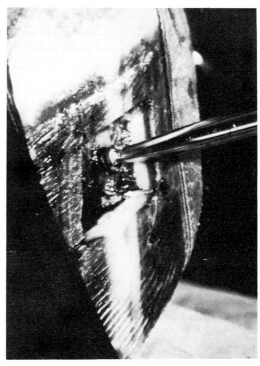

Broken pedal bone screwed together, during and after operation

Fracture of pedal bone healed one and a half years after the operation

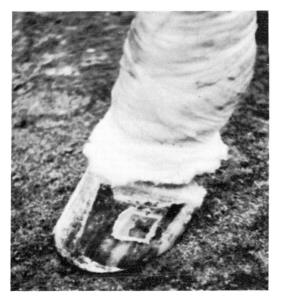

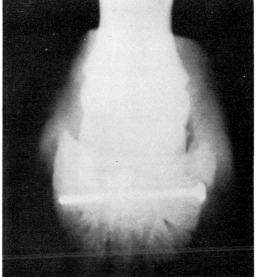

Fractures of the pedal, short pastern and long pastern bones and of small bones in the fetlock, knee, stifle and hock joints can often be treated successfully. Sometimes the fracture is screwed up and sometimes the fractured piece is removed.

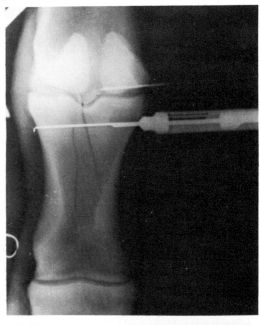

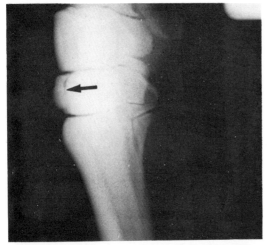

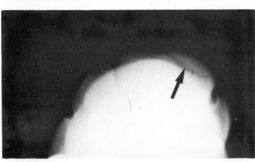

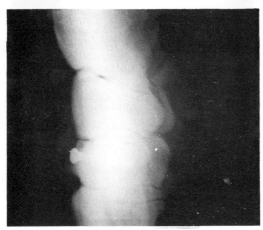

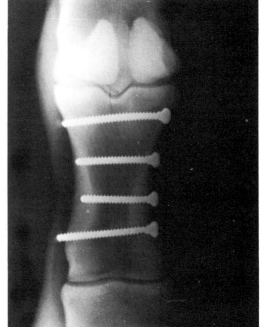

Fracture in knee joint before and after operation

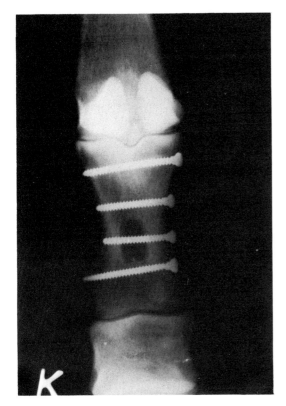

Fractured long pastern bone during and immediately after operation, and after six months

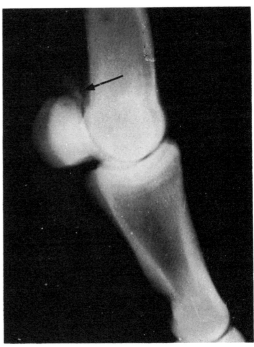

Fracture on top of sesamoid bone

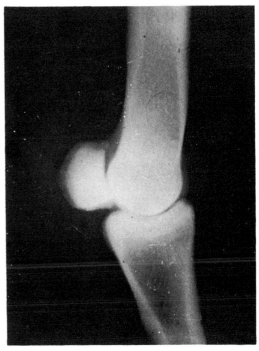

The fractured piece removed

Periostitis (inflamed bone membrane) and exostosis (growth of new bone), the latter a consequence of the former, are common causes of lameness. A blow or a cut can damage the membrane covering a bone, leading to a very local reaction, but more frequently the periostitis is more general, though most pronounced in the membranes of the radii and cannon bones in the fore-legs. An affected horse will often be very sensitive to pressure in these areas, and often new bone growth (exostosis) develops, some-times widespread, sometimes of limited extent.

If exostosis is X-rayed at the acute stage a very ragged and broken surface is revealed, becoming smoother and more level as the horse recovers. Horses with sore cannon bones move very stiffly and exhibit varying degrees of lameness. The most common sufferers from these conditions are horses being trained as show-jumpers and for dressage events; race-horses in training for a race; and two-year-olds and younger trotters in the earlier stages of training for racing. Often the rider or driver will notice a slight stiffness increasing every day, so that it takes longer to get the horse warmed up. In a serious case the horse will become tired and listless, and if it is trained or worked too hard it will lose its appetite and its muscles will start to atrophy. A skilful trainer or rider will notice these symptoms in time and alter the horse's training programme accordingly. All too often a horse's training is crammed into a certain period, instead of the horse being raced when it is ready. Each horse's training programme should be designed individually, taking into account its heredity, physical development, environment, feeding etc.

In less serious cases of periostitis light blistering and lighter work for a few weeks should be sufficient.

An acute case of periostitis will need a very long convalescence, sometimes as long as four or five months. The horse should be given exercise, pain-killers and general anti-inflammatory treatment.

Ragged new bone growth (exostosis) which is causing lameness, which may be on either or both sides of the bone, will need pin firing and rest for two months. Occasionally exostoses have to be removed. Given time, all horses with these conditions can be cured. Sore shin is the classical name for periostitis on the fore cannon bones of 2-year-old thoroughbreds. The inflammation is so severe that the cannon bones bulge forward. The treatment is the same as for other types of periostitis without exostosis.

Purulent ostitis and periostitis as a result of a wound require surgical treatment. Sometimes dead bone tissue must be removed, followed by a long course of antibiotics.

Dislocation or luxation as the result of a serious accident can affect any joint. The commonest dislocations are of the pastern and fetlock joints, the hock and the hip joints.

Serious dislocations will result in extensive damage to the tissues, with the ligaments giving way and the synovial membranes and the cartilages torn and crushed. Even if the dislocation can easily be reduced, the horse will be seriously crippled for life. Sometimes a horse can have the joint fixed permanently in one position so as to become usable for breeding purposes.

Subluxation or partial dislocation of the pastern joint is most frequently seen in Thoroughbreds and trotters. In its most usual form it does not cause lameness and does not appear to affect the horse's function. The cause is unknown.

Joints with wounds with or without infection are serious conditions requiring specialist attention as soon as possible.

A very insignificant wound penetrating a joint can cause the death or permanent crippling of a horse if it remains untreated. A period of several months' convalescence may often be needed after the wound has healed.

Metastatic inflammations of the joints, ie when bacteria are transported to one or several joints via the bloodstream from a focus of infection elsewhere in the body, are fairly common and are often not noticed in the early stages. The most classical of these infections (joint-ill) affects foals as the result of infection spreading through the bloodstream from the navel and entering the joints. Joint-ill in foals can, if noticed and treated in time, be cured completely if the available antibiotics are effective against the bacteria causing the infection.

Foals with joint-ill have a raised temperature, swollen joints, and have difficulty in getting up and in moving. They must be helped to suckle.

Other metastatic inflammations of the joints may be caused by infections such as strangles, inflammations of the lungs and throat, disorders of the gut, etc.

Unfortunately it is not always possible to locate the focus of the infection. Often when a sample of the synovial fluid is drawn off it proves impossible to grow any bacteria in the sample, even though they are present in inaccessible parts of the affected joint. In that case one has to try various types of antibiotics, starting usually with penicillin. Infected joints are always extremely painful, so a pain-killer will also be necessary.

Sprains are commonly diagnosed when a horse goes lame, but they are not as common

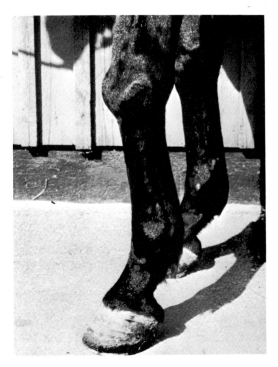

Inflammation of the knee causing deformation combined with bandy legs

in reality. The classical symptoms are sudden lameness, heat above the joint and extravasion (escape of fluid into the tissues) within the joint. If a joint low in the leg is sprained, a characteristic symptom is a throbbing pulse in the leg. In very serious cases blood will be found in the synovial fluid.

The treatment consists of cooling the sprained joint, careful exercise and pain-killers. In serious cases the fluid must be drained and the joint supported by an appropriate support bandage or plaster cast.

A horse which has been lame as a result of a sprain should be given a rest from its normal work for at least fourteen days and in most cases given cautious exercise. The joints most likely to be sprained are the fetlocks, both fore and hind.

An acute sprain of the pedal joint results in marked symptoms such as pronounced lame-

103

ness (grades 3–4) when trotting, swelling at the coronary band, a throbbing pulse in the leg and blood in the synovial fluid. The fluid should be tapped and drained off and pain-killers and anti-inflammatory treatment given.

At least two months' convalescence is necessary. This injury is not infrequently accompanied by a fracture of the pyramidal structure of the pedal bone.

Arthritis can be a complication following the wounds, infections and sprains mentioned above, but can also develop as the result of such causes as overwork, inadequate feeding, infestation by internal parasites, and allergies. There may also sometimes be an hereditary predisposition.

It is common to differentiate between *serous* and *osteo* arthritis. In the former the increase in the amount of synovial fluid (articular windgall) is a prominent symptom. In the latter the dominant symptoms are hard bony deposits around the joints and defective cartilages. Lameness is usually present, but large windgalls and large bony deposits (exostoses) can be present without lameness.

A young horse that is put to work too soon may often have windgalls for a while both in the joints and the tendon sheaths, until it becomes accustomed to the work.

Serous arthritis with lameness and an increase in the amount of synovial fluid is most often seen in the pedal and fetlock joints, the middle joint of the knee (carpus) and the shoulder joint in the fore-legs. The most commonly affected joints in the hind-legs are the fetlock hock, stifle and hip joints.

Serous arthritis of the pedal joint is characterised by a double-action step and swelling around the coronary band. The first step is to fit surgical shoes. Trotters are fitted with special pear-shaped shoes, others with a shoe with a short toe and side-clips. The amount of rest needed varies; some horses can carry on as usual, others may need a complete rest for two months or more. A little light blistering around the coronary band is also usual.

Serous arthritis of the fetlock joint is at present perhaps the most common cause of lameness in trotters, both in the fore- and hind-legs. Ingvar Fredricson's studies using a high-speed camera have revealed the strains to which a trotter's fetlocks are exposed on tracks with inadequately banked corners.

Treatment varies from case to case, depending on what the horse is used for and how long it has been lame. Usually anti-inflammatory treatment, both local and general, is prescribed, together with either a complete rest in a loose box or a little very cautious exercise.

Lameness caused by arthritis in the knee at the central carpal joint is an interesting condition that occurs in all types of horses, the cause of which we unfortunately do not know. It is met with in two- and three-year-old trotters, Thoroughbreds and in rather older saddle horses. At present it can only be diagnosed by a direct injection of an anaesthetic into the joint. Radiography does not show it. Typically this lameness increases as a result of work. Treatment consists of complete rest and injections of cortisone, hyaluronic acid etc direct into the joint.

Recovery takes at least two months, often as long as a year, but most horses will recover in time. In general they will not recover unless treated.

Serous arthritis of the shoulder joint is often passed over as a cause of lameness. It is, after all, not very common. It can only be diagnosed by anaesthetising the joint. Treatment is to inject cortisone into the joint once or several times and to rest the horse for two months or more.

Serous arthritis of the hock joint or bog spavin is encountered in all types of horses during immaturity. Inadequate or omitted worming, mineral deficiencies, or perhaps most frequently fodder too rich in protein will cause this condition; sometimes it may be caused by osteochondrosis (loosening of the epiphyses or growth plates) in the joint.

The horse is almost never lame. The swelling or swellings – they are often on both sides of the joint – can be quite considerable. First of all the causes must be eliminated by a regular worming schedule, a balanced ration and suitable exercise. If the cartilage has loosened to any extent an operation should be considered.

If the spavins are of long standing they may be tapped once or several times with an interval of a few weeks. At the same time cortisone is normally injected. If the deficiencies have been corrected the spavins normally diminish, but can take a long time, up to a year or even more. Sometimes the spavins will remain throughout the horse's life, often without inconvenience.

Serous arthritis of the stifle joint is becoming increasingly common both in immature horses of all types and in trotters competing in races.

The horse is likely to be lame, with a break in its stride, windgalls at both the patellar joint and the lateral condyle, together with a weakening of the extensor muscles of the knee.

A fairly frequent cause in young horses is separation of fragments of bone (osteochondrosis or 'joint mice') in the stifle joint.

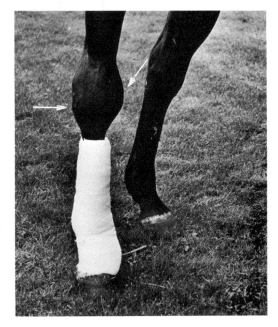

Bog spavin

In the latter case radical surgery to remove loose or loosening bone is necessary. In other cases the windgalls are tapped and cortisone or something similar is injected into the various parts of the knee joint. Complete rest is vital, for a minimum of two months.

Upward fixation of the patella is when the patella or knee-cap locks for a moment or for a longer period on the trochlea (central ridge) of the femur. The leg becomes completely stiff with rigid joints. Usually the patella 'clicks' quickly back into place. Young horses are most affected, particularly in the autumn when they have been out to grass for longer than usual, and are in poor condition because of the poor quality of the grazing. Upward fixation of the patella is also sometimes seen during convalescence.

If this condition becomes chronic, an operation is necessary. The medial patella ligament is cut, preferably on both legs with a week's interval. The operation has a very good chance of success. Convalescence takes

105

about six weeks, during which period the horse should be given a little gentle exercise. Many horses of various types have been operated on for upward fixation of the patella and gone on to be prize-winners in dressage and race-winning trotters. If a horse with this condition seems in poor condition, it is worthwhile trying to improve the diet and giving a series of vitamin B injections before resorting, if necessary, to the operation.

Serous arthritis of the hip joint is a condition often passed over in examinations, which only the highly-qualified specialist in lameness can diagnose, and then only by a process of elimination using direct injections of anaesthetics into the deep-seated hip-joint. Treatment is to inject cortisone direct into the hip joint at two-week intervals and to rest the horse for two months.

Osteo-arthritis is a dry inflammation of the joints. Its causes are frequently not understood; an infected joint or a bad sprain may start it off, but in many cases it develops very gradually. The most typical forms of osteo-arthritis are ringbone and bone spavin.

Ringbone is a term used of arthritis in the pastern joint. One form is typical of growing horses, thought to be associated with rapid growth, with symptoms very similar to those of rickets. It is also seen frequently in adult saddle horses.

Both types are characterised by hard, bony deposits (exostoses) around the pastern joints. Radiography reveals exostoses at the edges of the joints and degeneration of the cartilages in the joints. In young horses cysts may be detected in the bone under the cartilages.

Ringbones in young horses can stabilise so that such a horse at four years old may be a useful animal, but its market value will be low and insurance may be a problem. True

ringbone – causing lameness – in adult horses is incurable with present methods, though cutting the nerve can render the horse useable for a while. Cases have been reported in which an operation to fix the joint in one position has been a complete success, though convalescence takes more than a year.

Ringbone can occur on both fore- and hind-legs. It is rare in trotters. Subluxation of the pastern joint can be mistaken for ringbone but is usually quite harmless (see p 102).

Bone spavin is an arthritic condition of the hock joint, affecting either the gliding or the hinge joints. It can occur in growing horses (see ringbone, above) or in adult horses of all types. The classical test is to induce lameness as a result of flexing the hock. Exostoses occur on the inner, lower front edge, together with atrophication of the muscles of the croup. Bone spavin often affects both hocks and can develop and be cured without causing

Ringbone

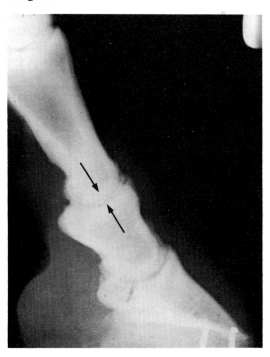

106

any lameness. Radiography will reveal deterioration of the cartilage in one, two or all three sections of the joint. If bone spavin is localised in the upper part of the hock joint the prognosis is poor.

Recovery occurs when the edges of the bones in the gliding joint grow together, ultimately fusing completely. This process can take more than a year. When the bones are fused there is much less pain.

A horse with bone spavin should be operated on if it limps. The operation enables the horse to be put back to work sooner but does not shorten the time needed for healing to take place. The horse should be exercised carefully throughout its convalescence.

Curbs and stringhalt also affect the hocks, though these are conditions unrelated to bone spavin.

Stringhalt is the name for a sudden snatching up of one or both hind legs while walking. The cause is quite unknown.

Stringhalt automatically disqualifies a horse for dressage or trotting. In some cases this habit may be corrected by peroneal tenotomy (cutting a tendon). If this fails the fault may possibly be cured by cutting the medial ligament as for upward fixation of the patella. In many cases absolutely nothing can be done. In some horses with incurable stringhalt a chronic inflammation of the spinal cord has been demonstrated.

Curbs are swellings at the back of the hock near the joint with the cannon bone. The cause is often an incorrect conformation. Trotters often have this fault. When a horse with this defect is trained (eg for racing) the deep flexor tendon reacts and the back of the hock becomes more swollen, hot and tender. Treatment is pin firing. Convalescence takes about six weeks.

Arthritis in the spinal joints and in the sacro-iliac articulation (between the pelvis and the

Bone spavin in middle gliding joint

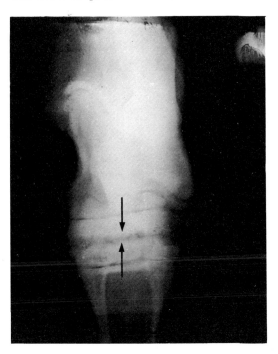

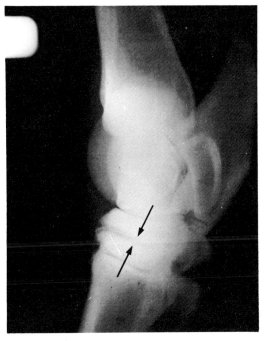

spine) occurs from time to time, but is very difficult to diagnose even with the most efficient X-ray equipment. The chief symptoms are pain in the back, muscular atrophication in the back and the croup, lameness in both hind-legs and, in certain cases where the pain is extreme, holding the tail higher than normal.

Treatment is rest, anti-inflammatory treatment, massage etc. Because diagnosis is so difficult the vet may tend to give very vague advice. 'Bone-setters' often have a great reputation for curing horses with back trouble, but if one has had the opportunity to study the wide variety of changes that can take place in the back as revealed by post mortem examinations one cannot but be very sceptical of claims that a layman with a mallet can knock the pain out of a horse's back!

Wobbler syndrome should also be described in this context. This refers to a horse with inco-ordinated movements (ataxia). It is, in other words, wobbly. The principal cause of wobbler syndrome is damage to the spinal column or the spinal cord.

Wobbler syndrome can be expected to arise when a group of young stallions is out to grass in a meadow. One day one of them is seen to be very wobbly but otherwise perfectly healthy. The reason is usually damage to the neck vertebrae causing pressure on the spinal cord. The young stallions have been fighting.

In a case like this the horse should be allowed to live for at least two months in case the injuries are temporary, in which case the unsteadiness decreases as time goes on. Within a year the inco-ordination is usually insignificant, only appearing when turning sharply and in a slight tendency to drag the feet. A horse with wobbler syndrome is often difficult to transport, as it finds it difficult to react to sharp turns or sudden halts. In some cases these horses can be ridden and driven in spite of their defect, but they never recover completely. A horse with wobbler syndrome that has not shown any notable improvement after two months should be destroyed.

Another type of wobbler syndrome that affects young horses is caused by an inflammation of the spinal cord, particularly its extremity, the cauda. In these cases the horse has suffered from a general infection originating in the respiratory tract some months before the wobbling symptoms appeared. This type of inco-ordination develops so gradually and is so mild that the layman is unlikely to come to the conclusion that it could be caused by an affection of the spinal cord. The prognosis is better in these cases, but one cannot be sure of success for about a year. All affections of the brain or spinal cord are very slow to heal.

BONE DISEASES IN YOUNG HORSES

Bone cysts in young horses occur in the pedal, short pastern, long pastern and cannon bones and in the small bones of the knee and the hock joints. They cause lameness and consist of cavities up to the size of a hazel nut in the bone tissue near to the joints. A bone cyst is connected by a narrow canal to the joint and the cartilage in the joint has an opening somewhat like a navel where the canal opens on to the joint. Anaesthetic injections into the joint stop the pain and the lameness ceases; in a while the cyst heals, but it can take more than a year. If the horse is allowed to rest and is not made to do any strenuous training until the cyst is fully healed it can be completely cured.

Bone cysts usually become established during the first year of life and are often overlooked during the diagnosis of lameness. They cannot be detected without radiography.

Joint mice (osteochondrosis) have become more frequent in recent years. They were once very common in foals and young horses of the Swedish Ardennes breed. Now they are often diagnosed in the stifle joints of young warm-blood horses and in the hock joints of young trotters. Occasionally something similar can be found in the fetlock joints. Fragments of bone, often of quite considerable size, become loose at the stifle joint and lie free in the joint cavity (joint

Cyst in short pastern

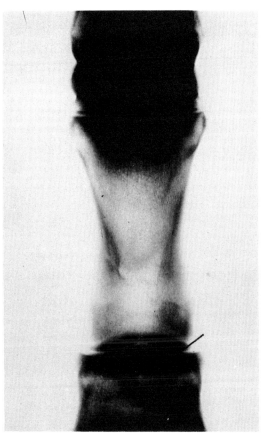

109

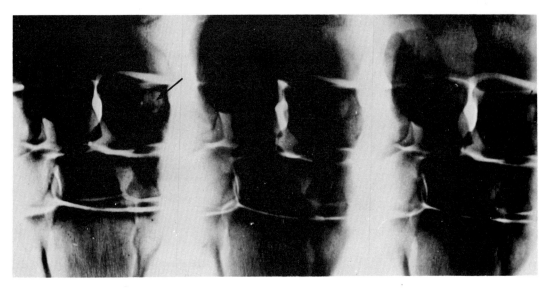

Cyst in knee (fore-leg)

mice). The synovial membranes react by producing increased amounts of synovial fluid, causing the development of a windgall. Lameness usually develops but need not be a permanent symptom. If the horse is to be retained an operation will be necessary to remove the joint mice. A lot of experience of this condition has been gained and the operation can be recommended.

The cause is unknown; similar conditions occur in humans, dogs and pigs, and one view is that the cause is very rapid growth. It may be that the cause is at least partly the changeover from natural foods such as hay and oats to various kinds of nuts.

Inflammation of the growth plates (epiphysitis) is not uncommon in young horses. Too much exercise on dry, hard ground, an inadequate diet and inadequate worming may be contributory causes. Young horses of 8–10 months exposed to these conditions will develop bony deposits around the ends of the bones near the joints, especially the fetlocks, but also the knees and more rarely the hocks. The affected horse becomes listless and stiff in its movements.

Radiography will reveal an inflammatory process going on in the upper growth plate on the long pastern and the lower growth plates of the cannon, radius and tibia. The elimination of any causes that can be demonstrated, improved rations, worming, extra vitamins and suitable exercise will usually succeed in restoring the growth plates to their normal condition. It is usually recommended that young horses that have had trouble with their growth plates should not go back into training until completely recovered. Progress should be checked by means of X-rays.

Horses reared from birth on artificial feeding-stuffs are more liable to inflammations of the growth plates.

WOUNDS AND DISEASES OF THE TENDONS

WOUNDS

A cure is almost impossible if an adult horse suffers from severed superficial and deep flexor tendons in either a fore- or a hind-leg. Sutures fail to hold the ends together, and the result is that the posture of the leg alters radically, with the fetlock sinking and the toe of the hoof pointing upwards.

It is questionable whether any treatment ought to be attempted in such cases, though there is a reasonable chance that foals can be cured and regain normal function.

If only part of a flexor tendon is cut or damaged the chances of recovery are better, although it will take a long time. Characteristically the affected tendon will swell along its whole length and become permanently thickened.

If the deep flexor tendon is completely severed in the region between the heels the chances of recovery and of regaining normal function are good. As well as normal treatment for a wound, including stitching, etc, a shoe with extra-long heels is fitted to counteract the toe's tendency to point upwards.

The extensor tendons can be more successfully treated than the flexor tendons. Even when an extensor tendon is completely cut and it is impossible to rejoin the ends with sutures, the tendon nevertheless becomes functional again and the knuckling-over resulting from the injury will eventually disappear. Treatment is to support the fetlocks with a suitable bandage until recovery is complete.

Rupture of the extensor tendons is fairly common in young foals, causing them to knuckle over. The rupture is inside the tendon sheath near the knee, where an escape of fluid (extravasion) will occur simultaneously. The foal will recover in a few weeks if the joint is supported with a bandage, and the position and function of the leg will return to normal.

Contracted tendons in foals which cause cocked ankles, and which do not respond to treatment with surgical shoes and lowered heels, are treated by cutting the tendons. This operation has so far given very encouraging results.

Contracted tendons in one- and two-year-olds develop very suddenly during the winter, causing the horse to hold the pasterns very upright on all four legs and tending towards more or less serious knuckling over. This condition seems to be completely untreatable and little is known about its causes. A young horse with this ailment will retain its upright pasterns and knuckling over for the rest of its life no matter how it is treated.

sometimes suffer from a chronic inflammation of the check ligaments of the deep flexor tendons of the fore-legs, without any apparent explanation. This condition is incurable and causes the horse considerable pain.

Bowed tendons appear mainly in two forms: an acute overstretching of a normal tendon

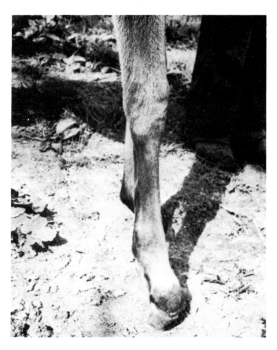

Foal with ruptured extensor tendon

Contracted tendons causing cocked ankle

Bowed or inflamed tendons. The tendons usually affected are the superficial flexor tendons on the fore-legs in racehorses, the superficial flexor tendons of the fore-legs in trotters, and less frequently in the hind-legs; and also the suspensory ligaments both fore and hind. Saddle horses most usually damage the superficial flexor tendons and occasionally the suspensory ligaments in the fore-legs. When horses were used for draught purposes they sometimes developed inflammations in the deep flexor tendons and in the lower branches of the suspensory ligaments in the fore-legs. Older retired horses of all types

is usually the result of an accident. According to the amount of strain to which the tendon has been subjected there may be torn tissue with some bleeding between the fibres, or sometimes single torn fibres or even complete rupture of the tendon. Minor less serious damage is most usual. This tendon damage is usually referred to as accidental.

The other main group begins with a gradual weakening of the tendon tissue as a result of intensive training and racing. Tendon cells and blood vessels degenerate, and eventually tissues rupture and bleeding occurs.

112

The first reactions in the tendon are often referred to as a 'warning'. The tendon develops a moderate swelling which is slightly warm and sensitive to pressure. Often when a horse has this kind of tendon damage without lameness training and racing is continued, but this only adds to the damage and the tendon swells more and more, until it may eventually rupture completely.

This type of damage to flexor tendons and suspensory ligaments is called fatigue damage and we owe our detailed knowledge of the process to work done more than forty years ago by Gerhard Forssell (1882–1964), one-time Professor of Surgery at the Swedish Veterinary Institute in Stockholm and perhaps the greatest equine orthopaedist the world has ever seen. The steeplechase jockey and research worker Berndt Strömberg has recently studied the biological changes that take place in fatigued tendons using modern angiographic techniques and with the help of thermal scanners. This fatigue damage affects mainly racehorses and trotters.

Accidental damage to tendons usually has a good prognosis, if the horse is allowed time to recover properly.

Fatigue damage to the superficial flexor tendons of racehorses can be treated in several ways, but whichever method is used the condition recurs in more than 50 per cent of cases. If the horse's racing career is broken off before too much damage has been done it can become a perfectly good saddle horse.

Fatigue damage to trotters has a better prognosis. In Sweden 75 per cent of operations on the fore suspensory ligament, 71 per cent of operations on the hind suspensory ligament, and 65 and 87 per cent of operations on the fore and hind flexor tendons respectively, are so successful that the horse can return to racing.

Tendon damage in saddle horses is rarely a serious problem. Acute cases should be given cold compresses changed every three hours, together with a course of anti-inflammatory injections or tablets. If the posture of the leg is affected and the fetlock sinks a support bandage should be put on.

The horse should be given a little careful exercise if possible, and after 48 hours a plaster cast or a gelatine–zinc oxide bandage put on and changed once a week. After about three weeks from the date of the injury, when all the acute swelling has disappeared, the leg should be blistered lightly. If the damage is primarily due to tendon fatigue an operation is indicated.

When a racehorse suffers from tendon damage it is always worth considering whether it would not be better both for the horse's well-being and the owner's pocket to re-train the horse as an ordinary saddle horse. This will reduce the convalescence needed to about two months. Convalescence after radical tendon surgery takes at least six months.

Rupture of the sheath of the superficial flexor tendon at the hock is a less common injury, mainly seen in Thoroughbreds, resulting in the tendon sliding outwards. Surgery seldom corrects it, and if the horse is allowed to live it cannot be used for anything except very easy riding or as a brood mare.

DISEASES OF THE TENDON SHEATHS AND BURSAE

Navicular disease is a chronic, slowly developing affliction of the navicular bursae of the fore-feet, often affecting both feet. Navicular disease in the hind-feet is very rare. Saddle horses often develop this condition, trotters almost never. A short, stumpy stride is characteristic, often leading the rider to suppose that the affliction is in the shoulder joint. A horse with advanced navicular disease turns on its hind-legs to take the weight of the body off the fore-legs. The fore-feet are put to the ground toes first.

If one fore-foot is anaesthetised the limp in the other becomes more pronounced.

Radiography reveals areas of rarefied bone in the navicular bone. The diagnosis of navicular disease must also take into account clinical observation of the typical symptoms. The cause is unknown, but contributory factors may be poor condition, insufficient exercise, being ridden at irregular intervals, so that the horse has long periods of activity followed by long periods of inactivity; if the horse spends a lot of time standing in a stall the disease will be greatly aggravated.

Cure is not possible, but surgical shoes with plastic soles, short toes and side clips can ease the horse's discomfort and postpone the development of permanent lameness, after which the only treatment that remains is neurectomy.

Inflammation of the tendon sheaths in the fetlock region, with windgalls varying in size and pressure, can cause lameness in both fore- and hind-legs. Tapping and draining the fluid and injections of cortisone etc can give good results. If the tendons inside are also damaged the prognosis is not so good. In some cases this condition is treated by pin firing. Recovery and convalescence take at least two months.

Extravasions (leakages of fluid) in the sheaths of the extensor tendons at the knee (fore-leg) of steeplechasers and showjumpers and under the skin at the inside of the knee in trotters should be treated as soon as possible after the accidents which cause them. If they are neglected chronic swellings will form which will possibly reduce the horse's usefulness. About ten days after an acute extravasion takes place it should be tapped and injected with a suitable medicament. Elastic support

bandages should be put on and the treatment repeated ten days later. Usually convalescence takes at least six weeks.

Capped elbow is an inflammation of the bursa at the point of the elbow caused by pressure and occurring most often when horses are housed in stalls with inadequate bedding. If the heels of the shoes are too long this can also contribute.

Recently developed extravasions should be treated with a cooling ointment (or similar treatment) and the cause must be eliminated. If the capped elbow is of long standing it should be treated as for other types of extravasion.

If a capped elbow becomes infected it should be treated surgically, but in general radical operative treatment is not recommended as recovery is likely to be slow and difficult.

Inflammation of the bursa of the biceps tendon at the point of the hock (*bursitis intertubercularis*) causes lameness and is apparently caused by an external injury to the point of the hock, eg a kick or a fall. Diagnosis is by means of local injections of anaesthetics. Treatment consists of repeated injections with a suitable cortisone preparation. The condition can be treated with much more chance of success since this drug became available. The horse should rest for at least two months.

Capped hock is a swelling of the (false) bursa under the skin at the point of the hock, often caused by horses knocking against the walls of stalls and loose-boxes or while being transported. Inadequate bedding and being housed in a stall increase the likelihood of contracting capped hock, which usually occurs on both hocks. Acute cases should be treated with a cooling ointment or similar preparation. Chronic cases should be tapped and drained. Occasionally the swellings contain loose particles, in which case surgical removal of these particles is recommended. Otherwise radical action is not recommended unless the swelling is infected.

Inflammation of the plantar bursa, which lies between the superficial flexor tendon and the Achilles tendon at the point of the hock, is an extravasion very reminiscent of capped hock, but which differs in that it often causes lameness.

Tapping the fluid and injections of enzymes and cortisone is the current treatment. Convalescence usually takes about two months. The chances of regaining full function are good so long as the superficial flexor tendon is not split where it crosses over the point of the hock. This is difficult to ascertain clinically.

Thoroughpin is an inflammation of the sheath of the deep flexor tendon at the hock causing swelling on both sides of the hock. Lameness is not usual; if the horse is not lame it may be ridden as usual. If it is lame the best treatment is to tap the fluid and give the

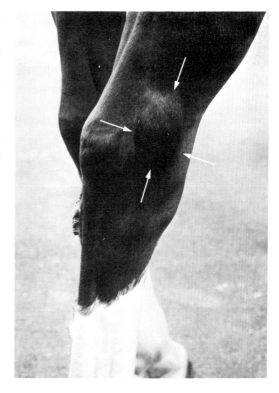

Hock with a thoroughpin

usual injections, in which case the horse should be allowed to convalesce for about two months.

DISEASES OF THE MUSCLES

'MONDAY MORNING DISEASE'

The best known of the horse's muscular disorders is Monday morning disease or 'setfast'. It was formerly a common affliction of heavy draught horses and generally appeared when a horse returned to work after a few days' rest. The cause was feeding the normal ration of concentrates when the horse was not working, leading to the storage of an abnormally high amount of glycogen in the musculature. When the horse was put to work the glycogen was broken down causing a build-up of lactic acid in the muscles. This led to widespread damage particularly to the muscles of the croup and thigh. The disease sometimes took a mild form, but not infrequently the horse became incapable of standing up; many horses were lost as a result.

Nowadays Monday morning disease occurs in racehorses. It is most common among trotters, but other racehorses and saddle horses are also affected. There are several causes; rest together with a carbohydrate-rich diet, and too little work, can have a certain significance. Research has also shown that horses have been subjected to stress (for example, transportation, change of surroundings or surgical operation) before the onset of the disease.

Arne Lindholm, who has done some fundamental research into this syndrome, divides it into three categories based on the symptoms and on enzyme analysis:

Mild Monday morning disease causes stiffness after work. The horse often scrapes the straw together with its fore-legs and moves its hindquarters as little as possible. The symptoms soon disappear, often without the owner having noticed anything.

Moderate Monday morning disease causes profuse sweating during work. In the loosebox the horse shows signs of moving with difficulty, and the musculature of the croup becomes hard and oversensitive. The symptoms recede within 3–4 hours.

Acute Monday morning disease. The symptoms appear after only 10–20 minutes' work. There is profuse sweating and pronounced stiffness in the hind-quarters. The horse's hind-legs sometimes develop a wobbly gait and the muscles are hard and tense. The symptoms in the hind-legs almost disappear after four hours but the gait may not return completely to normal for several days. The disease is most reliably diagnosed by taking a blood test to demonstrate the accumulation

116

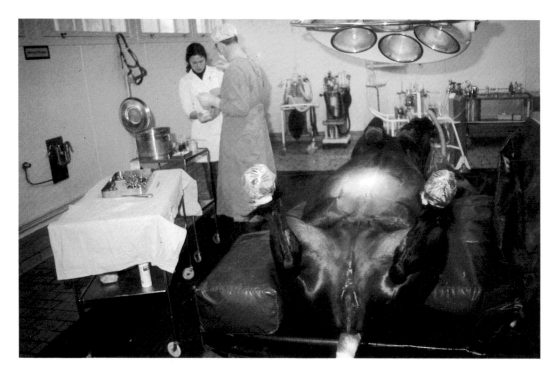

Preparing for a caesarean section

Birth of a foal by caesarean section

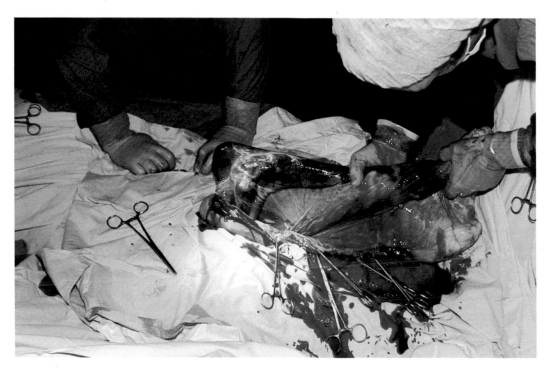

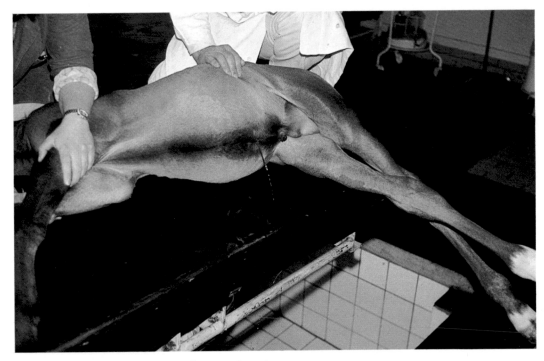

Foal with ruptured bladder. Note the pear-shaped abdomen. The urine is tapped and drained out of the abdominal cavity

Foal with scrotal hernia

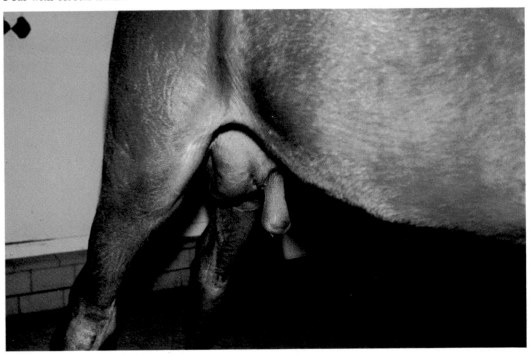

of the enzymes CPK and SGOT. Repeated blood tests will show when the horse is fit to work again. Treatment consists of medication with selenium, vitamins E and B, and rest. Adjustment of the ration when a horse is resting is important. The disease tends to recur.

GENERAL MUSCLE INFLAMMATION IN FOALS

Foals sometimes suffer from a serious muscular disease which can be fatal. The disease seems to appear within limited geographical areas. Some years ago there were several cases in southern Sweden. The same spring a number of young foals fell ill on a stud-farm in Denmark. The symptoms are a general stiffness in the muscles; the foal finds it difficult to rise and must be helped to its feet; the muscles in the back and croup and in the legs are hard and tense. The foal has difficulty eating because even the muscles of the jaw are affected. The crest is often swollen and sensitive. Breathing- and heart-rate are raised. The urine becomes red as a result of the colouring matter in the muscles being voided in the urine when the muscle fibres break up.

The cause of this disease is thought to be a diet lacking in selenium and vitamin E. Infections can also cause general inflammation of the muscles in foals. Treatment consists of supplying selenium and vitamins E and B. In a mild case the foal will recover, but acute cases lead to death or invalidisation. Keep the foal still while it is suffering from the disease, or the muscle damage will be made worse. Where this disease is prevalent the pregnant mare should be given preventive treatment in the later stages of pregnancy.

Foal with general muscle inflammation

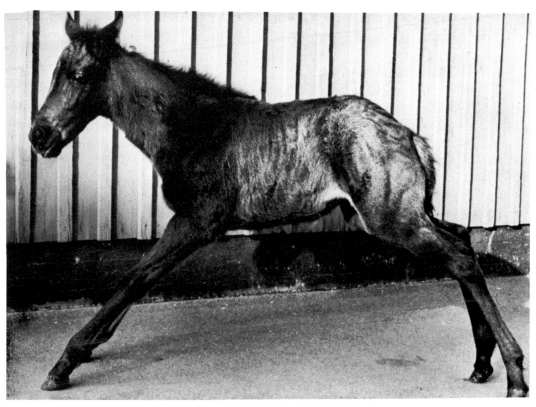

LAMENESS CAUSED BY DISEASES OF THE NERVOUS AND CIRCULATORY SYSTEMS

Wobbler syndrome has already been mentioned, p 108.

Nerve damage. A serious blow on the shoulder can damage the nerve which runs alongside the point of the shoulderblade. As a result the muscles which connect the shoulder to the chest cease to function and the shoulder 'falls away' from the chest when the horse moves. Recovery is possible, but it can take anything from 3–4 days to a year or more. In half the cases there is no recovery.

The nerve plexus below the shoulder can also be damaged as the result of a bad fall or if the horse has to lie on its side for many hours on an operating table. A horse with this kind of nerve damage is unable to move the limb affected. It perspires and shows obvious signs of pain. Within three or four days the lameness usually recedes.

Contusions in the nerves at the fetlocks can be caused by a horse rubbing itself. Severe pain causes a sudden limp which soon gets better. If these nerve contusions are repeated day after day a neuroma (nerve tumour) causing permanent pain may develop, in which case an operation will be necessary.

Iliac thrombosis is a disorder caused by blood clots in the arteries in the pelvic region affecting the hind-legs. The disorder may be anything from mild to very acute. Typically the horse moves perfectly normally when taken out of the stable. After being exercised for a while it begins to limp in one or both hind-legs, depending on the extent of the blood clots in the blood vessels. If one keeps the horse in motion it starts to sweat and to show marked symptoms of pain, while the lameness in the hind-legs becomes worse and worse. The reason for the development of these blood clots is unknown. When the disorder is discovered the clots are already 'organised' and scarcely treatable. When only a few smaller blood vessels are affected it is possible for other blood vessels to adapt themselves in the course of time and take over the function of the affected blood vessels.

DISEASES OF THE DIGESTIVE SYSTEM

TEETH

It is possible to determine a horse's age by examining its front teeth to see which are present and how much the surfaces have worn. To examine the condition of the teeth one parts the jaws using a ladder gag or a wedge-shaped mouth gag; examination is

Examining a horse's teeth

usually by palpation using one hand. Sometimes a mirror is necessary, sometimes also X-rays.

With the hand one checks the number of teeth and their positions in the jaws. It is important to note any gaps between the teeth. Both the grinding surfaces and the sides of the teeth should be palpated, and also the jaw-

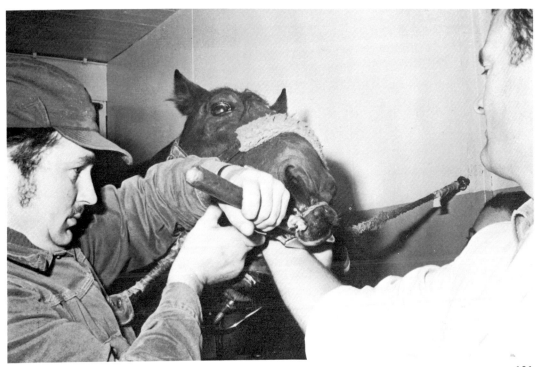

bones and mucous membranes. Unpleasant-smelling food residues should be noted. Horses are usually good-natured, and it is a simple matter to put on a ladder gag; but it is a dangerous instrument that, if used carelessly, can seriously injure the patient, the vet or his helpers. It may be necessary to give a horse a tranquilising injection before examining or treating teeth.

CONGENITAL DEFECTS

Overshot jaw and **undershot jaw** alter the way in which the teeth wear. The front teeth will not wear at all; with an undershot jaw the front premolars of the top jaw and the back molars of the lower jaw will develop sharp projections, and vice versa in cases of overshot jaw. Even in quite noticeable cases

Wedge gag and ladder gag

of over- and undershot jaw (which are really malformations) horses are able to obtain food and to maintain good condition.

Extra teeth (supernumerary teeth) may occur as extensions of rows of teeth or to one side of them. Extra cheek teeth are very common in trotters (wolf teeth) in front of the row of ordinary teeth in the cheek of the upper jaw. Trainers usually prefer to have this tooth removed as it is thought to cause the horse discomfort when the bit is put in.

Other types of supernumerary teeth are fairly rare. They can lead to cuts in the mouth or to tooth decay as the result of collecting impacted food residues.

Dental cysts can sometimes reach gigantic proportions, causing breathing difficulties and

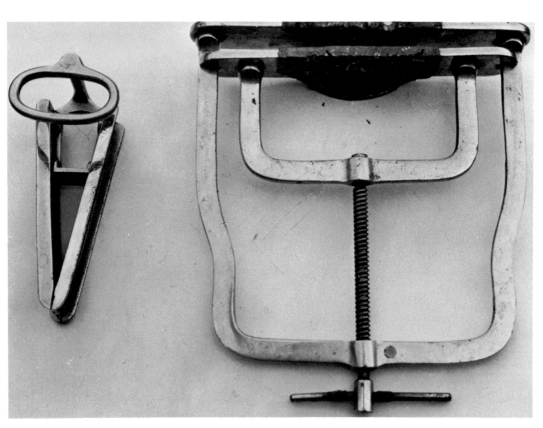

swellings in the region of the upper jaw. Sometimes foals and young horses suffer from these cysts. They must be removed by a radical (and often very difficult and bloody) operation.

Congenital fistulae in the ears are actually caused by a defective tooth root developing at the base of the ear and causing a fistula. The discharge from the ear will cease if the defective tooth is removed.

ACQUIRED DEFECTS

The commonest problem, which affects practically all horses when they lose first teeth, involves the development of sharp edges on the cheek teeth. This occurs on the outside of the upper jaw and the inside of the lower jaw, and is caused by inadequate sideways movements of the jaws while chewing.

Horses are made quite uncomfortable by the process of losing milk teeth and growing permanent teeth. The grinding surfaces tend not to wear down evenly at this period, and sharp edges develop. Horses' teeth grow continuously, distinguishing them from such animals as man, dogs and pigs, so that the rate of growth from the roots parallels the wear on the grinding surfaces. When the horse chews its food it chews 40–50 times on one side of the mouth, for perhaps 5 minutes, and then normally starts to chew in the same way on the other side of the mouth. Sharp-edged teeth cause cuts to the mucous membranes in the mouth. The horse becomes

Dental instruments: forceps and rasp

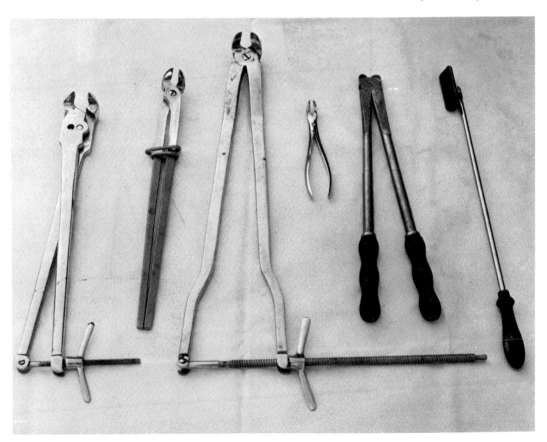

unwilling to eat and unwilling to chew food properly. As a result the sharp edges become even more pronounced and the horse's condition and performance begin to deteriorate.

Treatment consists of filing down the edges with a dental rasp.

Persisting milk teeth should be mentioned here as they often cause the development of these sharp-edged teeth. The milk teeth remain as caps on the permanent teeth as they grow, and remains of fodder can become packed between them, causing caries (tooth decay). This is easily diagnosed, and it is a simple matter to remove the milk teeth.

There are quite a variety of similar conditions from which horses may suffer. If a tooth is missing the corresponding tooth in the opposing jaw will become too long, with sharp points. These teeth must be brought down to the level of the other teeth at regular intervals. If this is neglected they will eventually become so long that they meet the gums in the opposing jaws, causing bone decay and severe pain. Sometimes abnormalities in the surfaces of the cheek teeth can be caused by the teeth being of varying degrees of hardness, which can cause *curved tables*, *step mouth* etc.

Shear mouth develops when the horse for some reason chews on only one side. The reason may be a painful chronic inflammation in one of the jaw joints, a chronic tooth defect, tooth decay, a broken tooth or a

Filing teeth, using a ladder gag

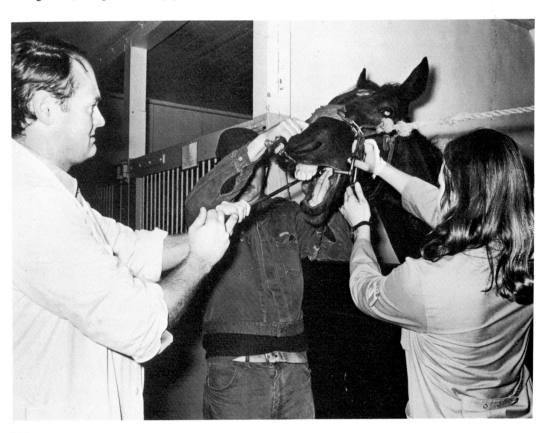

124

tumour on the jaw. As a result the teeth grow out and eventually come to resemble the blades of a pair of shears on the side that the horse does not chew with. The cause must first be treated and the level of the teeth reduced. The prognosis is poor, because the cause is often untreatable.

Tooth decay occurs in horses, though seldom in trotters. The most common causes are *impacted food residues*, *open pulp canals*, or a *fracture* or *crack* in a tooth. Impacted food residues only cause trouble as a rule in horses born with gaps between certain cheek teeth. Particles of food are pressed into these gaps during chewing; they start to decay, causing both bacterial and chemical attack of the tooth and the jaw bone. If a pulp canal is open food residues are packed into it in the same way. In this case the tooth is attacked from inside; the process often penetrates down into the root of the tooth, causing an abscess at the point of the tooth root, and often also attacking the actual socket in the jaw bone. If the affected tooth is in the upper jaw the abscess breaks through into the maxillary sinus, causing the cheek to swell, and the horse develops an unpleasant-smelling discharge from one nostril.

Teeth with caries in the pulp canal crack or break very easily. A fracture can be the cause of tooth decay, but this is less common.

The symptoms of tooth decay are reduced food intake and 'cudding' – taking up food, chewing it for a while and then dropping it out of the mouth again. Examination of the mouth reveals smelly food residues between

Filing teeth, using a wedge gag

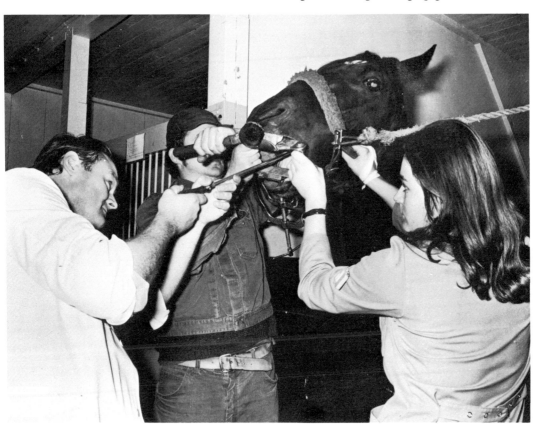

the affected teeth. A dental mirror will often help in assessing the nature of the decay; often radiography will be necessary to localise the decayed teeth.

The treatment is to remove the cause of the decay. If food is impacted without any very serious decay affecting the jaw bone, the crown of the tooth next to the gap must be cut away at the gum, the impacted residues removed and the wound disinfected. Usually the result is satisfactory. It is important to reduce any sharp overgrowth on the tooth opposing the site of the decay.

Root abscesses. If an abscess forms at the root of a tooth or if the whole tooth is seriously decayed or perhaps broken extraction becomes necessary. It can be done using large dental forceps but usually the tooth must be cut out with a mallet and dental chisel. If a tooth has been removed by an operation via one of the sinuses healing may take 4–5 months, but the result is usually very satisfactory.

In old age the teeth become very smooth. The ridges of enamel are worn completely away and the surfaces lose their grinding power. Horses with poor-quality teeth can develop this condition when still relatively young. Such horses need a diet that does not require too much chewing. The teeth of old horses sometimes become loose. This should be noticed so that very loose teeth can be extracted.

Tumours sometimes develop from the roots of one or more of the front teeth. This condition has only been observed by the authors in one- and two-year-old trotters. Lifting the horse's upper lip reveals one or more granular, conical, ulcerated growths that look malignant. They are in fact fairly undifferentiated odontomata. They are easily removed and have no tendency to recur. This naturally causes defects in the teeth concerned, but this doesn't seem to do any harm.

Cancer in the tooth sockets is by no means uncommon in older horses. The jaw swells slowly, and examination of the mouth reveals one or more teeth loosening in the growing tumour. The well known trotter 'Nancy Gay' suffered from this disease, and in spite of all that could be done for her it was not possible to prolong her life enough for her to be able to give birth to her last foal.

Regular dental care is an integral part of modern, rational horse-keeping. From 1½ to 6 years old, a horse's teeth should be inspected at least twice a year, for the reasons given above. Older horses should only need an annual inspection, unless for some reason they need to be treated more often.

Ageing horses should not be forgotten; their teeth may also need attention.

COLIC

Constipation. Colic refers to abdominal pain; this is most often caused in horses by constipation or blockage of the large intestine or the appendix.

There can be various causes of colic. Too abrupt a change from one type of fodder to another can cause an attack; constipation is common when horses are first fed in the stable after coming in from the summer grazings. Mouldy hay and rotten straw can be contributory causes. The symptoms are listlessness; uneasiness; a tendency to scrape with the fore-hooves; lying down, rolling and staring at the abdomen. The pulse-rate is moderately high, around 60 beats per minute, and the temperature is normal.

Diagnosis is by *per rectum* examination. The treatment is fasting, with about 4–5 litres of liquid paraffin per day, given by stomach tube in the case of an adult horse. If the horse is dehydrated fluid replacement will be necessary. Sometimes the blockage will not be loosened for three or four days. If the horse is in much pain it should be given painkillers intraveinously 2–3 times a day.

Colic of this type can be prevented by feeding with fresh fodder, making changes of fodder gradually, and regular exercise. When horses return to the stables after grazing all summer it is a good plan to give each horse 200g of molasses every day.

Meconium retention in new-born foals is usually released by an enema, or in mild cases by Microlax. Often oral dosing of liquid paraffin or castor oil is also necessary, together with fluid into the bloodstream if there is any risk of dehydration. Occasionally an abdominal operation may be necessary. Sometimes the small colon may be full of rubbery plugs which cannot be removed without actually massaging the intestines. Sometimes during this type of operation the cause will be found to be a malformation of the intestine – part of the intestine is quite simply missing. In such cases surgery is likely to be successful. Sometimes six-month-old foals can suffer from a type of constipation caused by a blockage in the small colon. Generally this can only be dislodged by direct massage, involving surgery. A massive invasion of intestinal parasites in the small intestine can cause blockages in foals, bringing about intussusception (see p 128).

Flatulent or tympanitic colic is caused by the accumulation of large amounts of gas distending the large intestines and causing the horse considerable pain. It often throws itself headlong on the ground and can soon inflict large abraded wounds on projecting parts of the body such as the ridges above the eyes, the elbows, the points of the croup, the knees, hocks and fetlocks. The abdomen becomes distended, and the pulse rises to 80–90 per minute. The cause may be rotten fodder, but more usually it is blood clots from the base of the aorta breaking free and passing into the smaller arteries supplying the intestines. This prevents the normal intestinal action and allows the gas to build up. The original blood clots in the aorta are caused by the activities of redworm larvae.

Flatulent colic can cause rupture of the stomach or of the part of the intestine with damaged circulation.

Treatment consists of emptying the gas and fluid in the stomach by means of a stomach tube. Often puncturing the gas-distended large intestine by means of a trocar is necessary. This is done through the left or right flank or both. This relieves the extreme pain, and anti-spasmodic drugs are also given.

In the early stages it is difficult to be sure about the chances of treatment being successful. It is important not to make hasty decisions before one is certain that the case is hopeless. On the other hand very careful nursing and continuous adaptation of the treatment to the development of the illness will be required if treatment is attempted.

The damage at the base of the aorta caused by parasitic larvae can heal in time, sometimes after or during several years, so that the attacks of tympanitic colic will cease in time. A daily dose of liquid paraffin is often to be recommended.

Intussusception (the telescoping of one part of the intestine into an adjacent part, causing blockage) is commonest in foals that have diarrhoea and is rare in adult horses. The condition affects the small intestine; usually in the adult horse the small intestine telescopes into the appendix.

The symptoms are usually those of mild colic, differing in that they do not respond to the normal colic treatment. Diagnosis is difficult, involving exploratory laparotomy. When the symptoms of inexplicable and worsening attacks of colic fail to clear up after 12 hours the abdomen is opened. The telescoped section of the intestine is either pulled straight or removed. The horse dies unless this is done.

Twist colic occurs in various forms and gives all the symptoms of violent colic.

Strangulated scrotal hernia. Twist colic also includes the trapping of the intestines in the scrotum in stallions. This is very common in American trotters and is called strangulated scrotal hernia. It can occur in horses of all ages.

Trotter foals are often born with scrotal hernia. Usually it disappears as the horse grows, but it can become trapped or strangulated. In adult stallions this often occurs after a training session. In addition to the normal symptoms of colic the horse has a swollen, painful scrotum. The condition must be operated on as soon as possible, and the stallion should be castrated at the same time and on both sides, no matter what his age. Otherwise the risk of a strangulated hernia remains on the other side. Stallions with this type of hernia, whether congenital or otherwise, should not be used for breeding.

The prognosis for this kind of colic is very good if it is detected and operated on in time; that is, within a few hours.

Other forms of twist colic include volvulus (a twisted small intestine) and volvulus mesenterialis, which is the name for a similar condition caused by a larger organ rotating on its suspending membrane, and also similar conditions in the large intestine. All give dramatic symptoms. The pulse rises to about 100 per minute, and the mucous membranes of the mouth, eyes and vulva become a blueish red. The horse sweats and the pain makes it ungovernable. Diagnosis is by means of a rectal examination. Gas-filled small intestines can now be felt lying in the abdomen like hard-pumped bicycle tyres. The abdomen is punctured, releasing fluid mixed with blood, but usually one has to resort to exploratory laparotomy for the final diagnosis. Unfortunately operations usually fail because of the difficulty of restoring the intestines to their proper places and the horse has to be destroyed. There are cases of twist that are operable if caught in time.

A horse with gut twist and violent symptoms suddenly becomes very quiet towards the end. This means that death can be expected within 5–6 hours; usually the stomach has burst and the general poisoning has suppressed the activities of all the vital organs and also the symptoms of pain.

Grass sickness should be mentioned here, as

it often results in symptoms very like those of colic as the result of secondary blockage of the large intestine. Grass sickness makes its appearance in certain years and in certain pastures 3–4 weeks after the horses are put out to grass for the summer. In Sweden the disease has been most prevalent on ground owned by Herrevad Abbey in Skåne, and at Utnäslöt near Strömsholm in Västmannland. The sickness has also been diagnosed in other parts of Skåne, for example in Kullabygden, in the region of Helsingborg and around Ringsjö. Grass sickness has also affected horses stabled for the winter.

About ten years ago five horses died of grass sickness in a stable near Malmö during the month of November. Investigations most notably by the Swedish professor of pathology Anna Lisa Obel demonstrated that the disease probably is caused by a virus; the disease attacks and to some extent destroys the nerve centres of the sympathetic nervous system of the thoracic and abdominal organs.

Grass sickness takes three main forms: a rapidly fatal, a slow-developing but fatal, and a chronic form from which the horse usually recovers.

All three forms begin with colic symptoms, sweating and pronounced muscular tremors. Blockage of the large intestine can be felt on *per rectum* examination. If a stomach tube is inserted a large amount (20–25 litres) of noxious fluid runs out of the stomach.

Death may occur suddenly and unexpectedly within a day or so or after several days or several weeks. Horses that survive

Chronic grass sickness

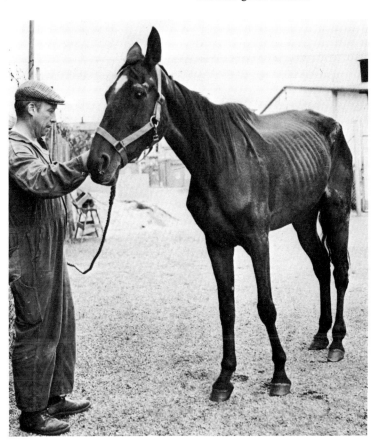

become very hollow in the abdomen and in general resemble greyhounds. It takes years for them to regain normal health but they never regain normal stamina. The only sure diagnosis is by post mortem examination. If it is a grass sickness year the experienced clinician will recognise the disease at once and recommend the only sensible course of action, ie slaughter.

Renal colic (due to kidney stones etc) is rare in horses. Many forms of colic caused by something wrong in the alimentary canal can also give the impression that the horse has difficulty in urinating. It stands and strains, but this usually has no connection with the urinary tract.

Part of oesophagus showing ulceration and narrowing that causes blockage

Colic caused by torsion of the uterus is included in the chapter on diseases of the genito-urinary tract.

BLOCKAGE OF THE OESOPHAGUS

Blockage of the oesophagus is very common nowadays. It can affect any horse fed with sugar-beet pulp that has not been soaked beforehand. The symptoms are quite characteristic. The animal is obviously distressed. Particles of fodder and saliva run from the nose and the horse holds its head low and dribbles. Sometimes the blockage in the gullet is visible as a lump low down on the left-hand side of the neck.

Quite often the discharge from the nostrils causes such a blockage to be mistaken for a sudden attack of strangles. If a stomach

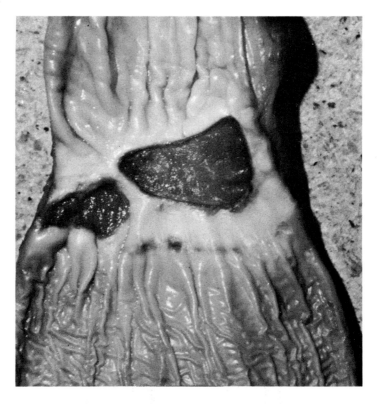

tube is inserted the blockage can be felt, most often in the region of the chest.

Treatment with one or more anti-spasmodic injections is sometimes sufficient, allowing the blockage to slide down into the stomach, but with more serious cases this treatment is inadequate, and the blockage has to be washed out. This should be done under a general anaesthetic, as it is very painful. It may take several hours to loosen the blockage, and breathing can easily be obstructed, so that it is usually necessary to insert a breathing tube into the windpipe. A simultaneous drop feed of large quantities of physiological saline solution is also necessary to counteract the inevitable dehydration of the tissues. Even in serious blockages of the oesophagus requiring very dramatic methods of treatment the outcome is usually successful.

When feeding horses on sugar-beet pulp, always take the precaution of soaking it beforehand.

Another type of oesophagal blockage is seen in foals and young horses with chronic ulceration of the mucous membrane of the oesophagus. This blockage occurs irrespective of the type of fodder and is localised above a ring-shaped ulcer several centimetres long. Nothing is known about the cause of this ulcer; it never heals and the horse loses weight because of repeated blockages, until there is no alternative but slaughter.

DIARRHOEA

Enteritis with diarrhoea is common in foals, often striking as early as their ninth day when the mare comes on heat after the birth. Frequently the diarrhoea remains after the mare is no longer on heat.

The foal is apparently unaffected, but its tail is kept wet by the thinnness of the faeces and the hair falls off the insides of the thighs. Both the mare's milk and the foal's faeces should be examined bacteriologically. While waiting for the results the foal should be given charcoal, a sulpha drug, streptomycin, chloramphenicol etc.

Acute enteritis with diarrhoea also affects adult horses. Unsuitable fodder such as mouldy hay and mouldy oats can cause it, as can viruses, bacteria, etc. Temporary accommodation for horses at gatherings such as race meetings with primitive and unhygienic stabling can lead to several horses being affected at once.

Salmonella can attack horses. Foals and adult animals with diarrhoea and a temperature should be examined for salmonella. About ten years ago at an agricultural show in the south of Sweden with a large animal section about ten foals went down with salmonella and several died. The cause was one of the foals having slight diarrhoea and in fact being infected with salmonella. All the horses at the show were drenched with sweat when they arrived because of a sudden heatwave,

and that night the weather suddenly became cold and rainy, making the foals less resistant. If salmonella is diagnosed the veterinary surgeon should be notified, and also if necessary the local public health authorities, who decide what measures must be taken.

Colitis. Racehorses, particularly trotters, can suffer from an inflammation of the large intestine (colitis) which can easily become chronic. Horses with colitis have loose, unpleasant-smelling faeces. Colitis is very difficult to treat. A carefully regulated diet, including soured milk, and medical treatment can help. Chronic colitis can cause the intestinal wall to become so thin that it suddenly ruptures, and the horse dies soon afterwards. It is thought that the stress of training and racing can be a contributory factor in the development of colitis. Horses fed with conventional fodders such as hay and oats very rarely suffer from this disease.

A related disease, thought to be caused by a sudden increase in one of the clostridium group of bacteria, whose toxins produce the very serious symptoms, develops extremely rapidly. An apparently completely healthy horse falls very suddenly ill, with severe diarrhoea and consequent dehydration. The animal is likely to die very quickly in spite of prompt and intensive treatment.

Stress is thought to play an important part in the very rapid development of this disease.

JAUNDICE

The liver is the largest gland in the body, and of great importance for excreting the toxic products which enter or are produced in the gut. These are absorbed by the blood, arrive at the liver in the bloodstream and are there broken down into harmless substances. Exhausted red blood corpuscles are broken down in the liver and changed into bile pigment which is discharged into the contents of the gut. Other important liver functions are connected with the circulation of carbohydrates and fats in the body. Proteins are transformed into carbohydrates or other proteins. The liver synthesises many substances that are very important for the bodily functions, such as bile, which makes possible the absorption of fats from the intestines.

Liver diseases often result in jaundice, which is a yellowing of mucous membranes best seen in the eyes, mouth and vagina. The urine becomes brownish yellow. The yellow colour is the result of an excess of bile pigments in the blood.

If the bile ducts are blocked by parasites or by tumours or because of inflammation, the result is jaundice. A common cause of jaundice is acute and prolonged blockages of the large intestine and appendix. When the blockages are released the yellow colour soon disappears from the mucous membranes.

If for various reasons the red blood cells are destroyed in large quantities, abnormal quantities of bile pigments are synthesised and these enter the blood and cause jaundice.

Among the diseases which cause destruction of the red blood corpuscles are such virus diseases as infectious equine anaemia and equine viral arteritis.

Jaundice in new-born foals. New-born foals sometimes have jaundice as a result of the mare developing antibodies against her own foetus. The antibodies are released into the colostrum mainly during the first 48 hours after the birth of the foal. The foal is born perfectly healthy until it begins to suckle, receiving a large quantity of antibodies. These are absorbed in the gut, entering the bloodstream and joining up with the red blood corpuscles, preventing them from functioning normally. The foal becomes anaemic, jaundiced and generally ill. The breathing- and heart-rates increase, the foal becomes weak and is unable to suckle.

The only way to save the foal is to give a blood transfusion while draining off an equal volume of the damaged blood, or in other words to replace the blood.

Preventive measures The disease can be avoided by preventing the foal from suckling the mare for the first 24 hours in cases where it is thought likely, in which case colostrum from another mare must be given to the foal instead. Colostrum from a cow can also be used. It is very important to milk the mare dry once an hour for the first 24 hours to free her milk of the antibodies.

A good piece of advice for horse-breeders

is to try to store a few litres of colostrum from a healthy mare in the freezer. This could save the life of a new-born foal that was unable for some reason to have its own mother's milk.

Poisoning. Jaundice can also be caused by various types of poisoning. These may be chemical poisons, or toxins released by infective agents which attack the tissues of the liver and hinder the breakdown of the bile. Chemical poisons may be arsenic, lead, copper, phosphorus, carbon disulphide and phenothiazine. Note that overdoses of worming preparations, which contain the two last-named substances, can cause jaundice in horses from time to time. Even certain plants, such as alsike clover, can if eaten in large quantities cause liver damage leading to jaundice and eventually to cirrhosis of the liver.

Poisoning can take various forms. Sometimes there will be symptoms from the brain and the spinal cord. The horse may become lethargic, support its head on a convenient object, go round in circles, lose co-ordination and become jaundiced. In advanced cases there may be little chance of recovery. If caught early recovery may be possible if the diet is corrected and tonics are given.

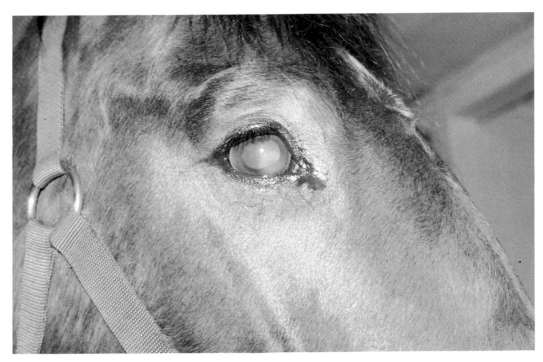

Inflammation of the cornea

If the cornea is damaged the third eyelid is
sometimes sutured across the eye to protect it
while the injury heals

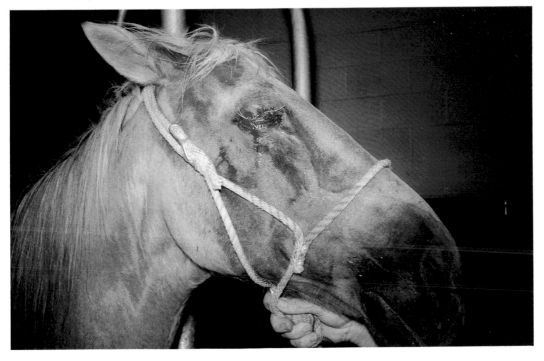

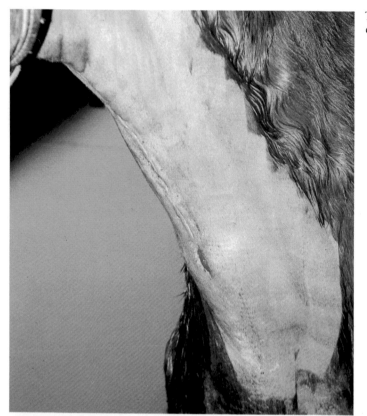

Three weeks after an operation to cure crib-biting

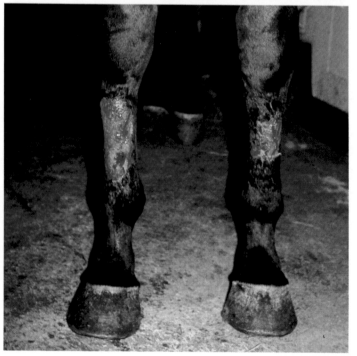

Horse treated with an 'Irish blister'

DISEASES OF THE RESPIRATORY SYSTEM

Nosebleed usually occurs in racehorses in connection with training or racing. Often there is a history of nosebleed in certain Thoroughbred blood-lines which is thought in such cases to be the result of fragile walls in the blood-vessels of the nose. Racehorses which suffer from recurrent nosebleeds during training or racing often suffer from some circulatory defect. It is not unusual to discover an inflammation of the heart muscle in these horses. Very dangerous nosebleeds can be caused by fungal infections of the guttural pouches. When the vet administers medicine by stomach tube or examines a horse with a laryngoscope very copious bleeding may be caused by the horse making a sudden jerk while being treated or examined. Such nosebleeds may look very unpleasant but the bleeding usually ceases after 10–15 minutes, or even sooner if the horse's nose is held up.

Coughing. Nasal discharges and coughing are symptoms originating in the upper respiratory tract. In acute cases the primary cause is most often a viral infection. Modern horses are exposed to a wide variety of viruses, which are continually being spread as a result of the extensive international horse trade and the interchange stimulated by racing both nationally and internationally.

Influenza viruses 1 and 2 and equine herpes-virus (virus abortion) are infections which cause inflammation of the nasal passages and the bronchi and lead to the development of nasal discharge, coughing and fever. The period of incubation is very short, sometimes as little as 48 hours.

The preliminary feverish stage may be over in 24 hours, often without having been noticed. After a few days the nasal discharge and coughing may start, but these symptoms often moderate and then disappear completely within a very short time.

The primary infection may be followed by secondary infections in which case the horse will become feverish once more, and the previously clear nasal discharge will become yellow and purulent. The submaxillary lymph glands become swollen and symptoms of pneumonia can also appear.

These developments are mainly seen in foals, which are more liable to develop pneumonia than adult horses. The congregation of mares with foals at stud farms during the breeding season provides one natural explanation for the high incidence of pneumonia in foals.

The course of the disease and the outcome depend entirely on the types of secondary infection that follow the primary virus disease. Thus if *Streptococcus equi* is present and causes abscesses in the submaxillary lymph glands and salivary glands, the disease will be referred to as strangles.

Bastard strangles is the name for the condition caused by the spread of the strangles to lymph glands elsewhere in the body, to the joints, the eyes etc.

Streptococcus equi has so far been very sensitive to penicillin, and treatment is therefore not usually difficult if the correct course of penicillin is given.

Secondary infections of another type and of a much more serious nature can also occur. Examples are the hemolytic staphylococcus and *Shigella equirulis* which are not affected by penicillin. Other antibiotics must be tried, but will often give very poor results.

Pneumonia in foals. A quite distinct form of pneumonia occurs in certain years in *two-month-old foals*. At first the foal's general condition is not affected; the first symptom is rapid and pronounced abdominal breathing. On examination the foal is found to have a somewhat raised temperature, around 39°C, rapid breathing and when the lungs are listened to both dry and moist râles can be heard. The causal organism was identified by the Swedish bacteriologist Hilding Magnusson and given the name *Corynebacterium equi*. It responds to certain types of

penicillin such as chloramphenicol, neomycin etc. If not checked in time these bacteria will cause widespread abscesses of all sizes. Often several foals will contract the disease on the same property in certain years. The first case is normally discovered too late, but increased vigilance and the timely use of antibiotics usually succeed in halting the outbreak, although the course of the disease can be very long drawn out.

It is not known why the disease occurs in certain years and not in others.

Routine precautions to be taken in the event of an outbreak of a respiratory infection

Isolate the infected stable. Horses should not be moved in or out.

Check the temperature of every horse every day.

Give only gentle exercise to horses with fever and other symptoms.

Good ventilation, dust-free feeding *and* dust-free mucking-out should be aimed for as far as possible.

Antibiotic treatment and chemotherapy should only begin if a secondary infection with a new fever begins, marked by a persistent nasal discharge and cough. The aim should always be to mobilise the animal's own powers of resistance before treatment begins. When treatment with an antibiotic or sulpha drug begins it should continue for at least seven days. To give an injection of penicillin once only is a serious mistake which may lead to the causal organism developing resistance to the antibiotic. If abscesses develop they should be lanced when they are ripe if they are at all accessible.

At the same time as antibiotic treatment

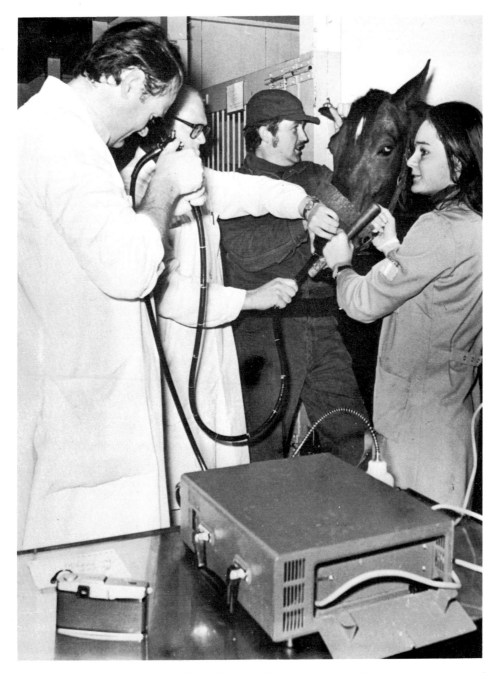

Examining nose, throat, larynx and trachea using a fibre-optic laryngoscope

is given it may be helpful to give phenylbutazone which will give a more effective penetration of the actual medicament.

Convalescence can only be decided on by considering the severity of the respiratory infection in a particular case.

Preventive measures are discussed in the chapter on infectious diseases, p 66.

COMPLICATIONS RESULTING FROM GENERAL INFLAMMATIONS OF THE RESPIRATORY TRACT

Sinusitis is quite frequent. A single- or double-sided nasal discharge with an unpleasant smell, and warmth and sensitivity around the frontal and maxillary sinuses are typical symptoms. Often an operation is necessary, which involves opening the sinuses.

Pharyngitis (inflammation of the throat) with follicular enlargement in the mucous membrane is common in young horses that are being trained. Diagnosis is by means of a laryngoscope, an optical instrument with which one examines the mucous membranes of the throat.

Such throat inflammations reduce the horse's capacity for work and sometimes cause râles when the horse breathes. Treatment consists of injections of sulpha drugs or antibiotics.

Inflammation of the guttural pouch is a rare occurrence. The guttural pouch (air sac) is a protuberance on the eustachian tube peculiar to the horse. The inflammation is often only on one side, causing a discharge from only one nostril. Diagnosis is made using a laryngoscope, and treatment is generally surgical.

In *young foals* these air sacs can become abnormally and pathologically full of air, which does not seem to cause them much discomfort but makes them look as if they have mumps. Treatment is surgical, and there is a risk that the condition may recur.

Tongue swallowing is a frequent complication

Chronic sinusitis with raising of frontal bone

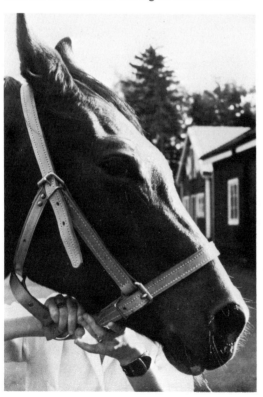

Horse after operation for purulent sinusitis

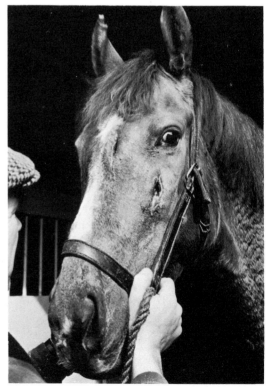

following pharyngitis in trotters and Thoroughbreds. The soft palate makes a characteristic 'clucking' sound during strenuous exertion and particularly when the horse is coming to a halt, and can obstruct the horse's breathing.

The weakened soft palate is shortened surgically and strengthened by diathermy (heat treatment).

Whistling is another complication following respiratory infection, although there may also be a constitutional disposition. It occurs in Thoroughbreds and warm-blood horses but very rarely in trotters or ponies.

Whistling is a noise which occurs when a horse breathes in and which is caused by paralysis of the left recurrent nerve which controls the movements of the vocal cords. The paralysed left-hand vocal cord is sucked in to the middle of the larynx, obstructing the flow of air and causing the very characteristic whistling sound. The paralysis can be so severe that the horse becomes incapable of any strenuous exercise.

Whistling can be cured by a surgical operation to remove part of the mucous membrane of the larynx; the vocal cords during healing take up a position in which they no longer obstruct the air flow. Usually the horse still makes some kind of noise even after the operation but the air passage is no longer obstructed and the horse is therefore capable of strenuous exercise. Healing and convalescence after the operation normally takes about six weeks.

Chronic bronchitis accompanied by a chronic or recurrent cough is the most common

Horse after operation to relieve purulent inflammation of the guttural pouch, and fitted with canulae to assist breathing

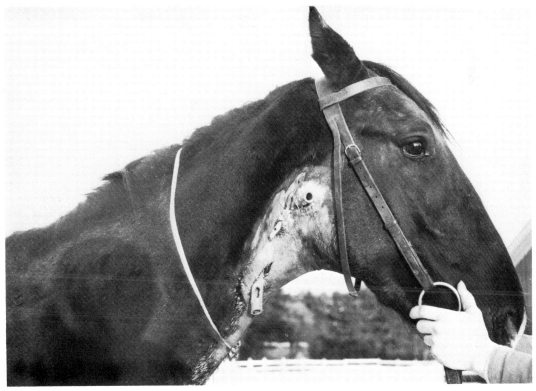

complication of all. A horse suffering from this condition may start to cough at the least exertion, so that it becomes impossible to ride or drive it. It often coughs in the stable, too, especially during mucking-out and feeding. If pressure is applied to the throat just below the larynx a series of coughs results. The horse exhibits pronounced abdominal breathing when at rest. After exercise a clear discharge is noticeable. Such horses can be nursed back to health, but it takes a long time and the treatment often needs to be finished off by a whole summer out to grass both day and night. Certain hygienic measures in the stable, such as good ventilation, and air with a suitable moisture content and free from dust especially during mucking-out and feeding, are essential, and it may be worth considering using shavings for bedding and going over to grass nuts instead of hay. Treatment is a long-term course of the appropriately tested antibiotic together with cortisone and the classical and modern relaxant and expectorant preparations.

Broken wind or chronic pulmonary emphysema is the incurable final phase of the preceding disease. The horse breathes rapidly, more than thirty times a minute, with a double flank action. The lungs are enlarged, and moist and dry râles can be heard.

Broken winded horses cannot do any work. Cortisone treatment may help when their breathing becomes very difficult, but such horses must eventually be slaughtered on humanitarian grounds.

Anasarca is a rare complication following strangles. Quite unexpectedly a horse that has previously had strangles is discovered to have extremely swollen legs and a swollen head that it can scarcely lift. In extremely severe cases fluid runs out through the skin both on the head and on the legs. The temperature is high, around 40°C, and the horse's general condition is poor.

It is believed that a focus of infection remaining in the body from the previous attack of strangles causes the widespread vascular damage which leads to accumulation of fluid in the tissues, particularly under the skin.

It is very difficult to assess the chances of recovery. Sudden heart failure is a possibility, but with the modern medical arsenal one can generally save the animal. There is a risk of recurrence.

HEART DISEASE

Considerable demands are made upon horses that take part in competitive sports, which makes it very important that the heart and the circulatory system in general should function perfectly. Such horses should be trained to do the work expected of them, but quite often they may be found not to be capable of it. The causes may be impaired lungs, anaemia, weakening muscles or a weak heart, for example. The heart is a powerful muscle, which by alternate suction and pressure makes the blood circulate through the body. An adult horse at rest should have a heart-rate of about 40–50 beats per minute. A horse in very good condition may have a lower heart-rate, while it may be higher in young animals. A horse making its utmost exertions can reach a heart rate of 250–300 beats per minute. If the heart is to be capable of withstanding such exertions it must be gradually trained, which causes it to expand and to develop a richer network of blood-vessels. It has been demonstrated that training must begin when a horse is 2–3 years old if its heart is to attain maximum capacity later in life.

The transport of oxygen. Transport of oxygen is of vital importance to the horse's performance. The red blood corpuscles take up oxygen as the blood passes through the lungs. The better the development of the lung tissues, the greater is their capacity to supply the blood corpuscles with oxygen. The oxygen-transporting capacity of the circulatory system depends upon the heart's ability to pump the blood round, the number of red blood corpuscles and the elasticity of the blood vessels. A high capacity to transport oxygen implies that a horse is very fit.

Training also implies that the muscles involved in the training exercises grow larger, develop a better blood-supply and hence a better supply of oxygen and nutrition, which leads to increased muscular stamina. Oxygen can be stored in muscle tissue to be used during extra exertion. Similarly, the capacity to store sugar in the muscles can influence performance, especially during prolonged muscular exertions. The conversion which takes place in the muscles in the presence of oxygen is aerobic conversion.

Energy can also be produced in the muscles in the absence of oxygen, which is referred to as anaerobic conversion. This occurs during short bursts of activity. The energy-rich substances which are broken down must be re-built, which requires oxygen. The physiology of modern horse training has been scientifically worked out by Professor Sune

143

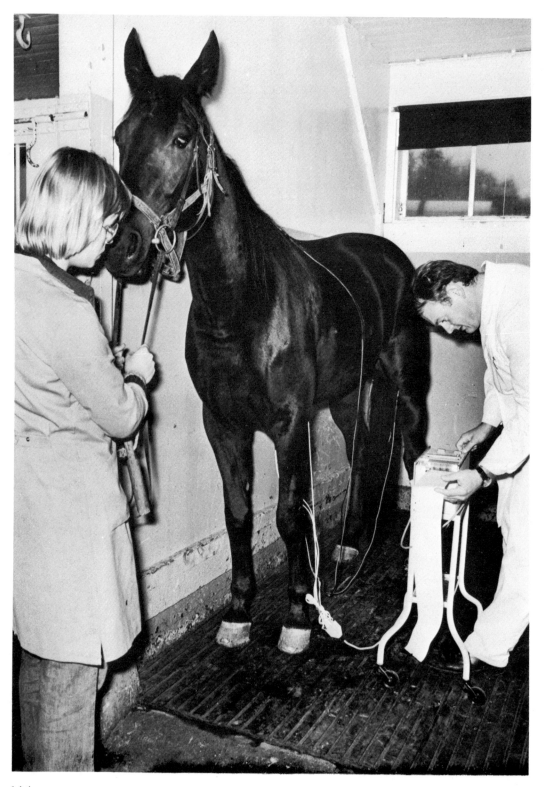

Persson and his colleagues at the Swedish Veterinary Institute.

EXAMINING THE HEART

The heart is listened to from both sides of the chest. Any changes of the heart's rhythm, frequency or sound are noted. This should be done both at rest and after exercise. Any suspicions are clarified by the use of an ECG examination. A special instrument – an electrocardiograph – registers the electrical charges which spread through the heart from the sino-atrial node, causing the heart to contract. Wires which are attached to various parts of the horse's body convey these impulses to a recording device which makes a trace on a sheet of paper. This trace is an electrocardiogram, which can be analysed.

Myocarditis (inflamed heart muscle). The ECG enables one to read off any changes in the rhythm and frequency of the heart and to decide whether the heart muscle is damaged. Damaged valves cannot be shown up by an ECG.

As mentioned above, inflammation of the heart muscle is a fairly frequent complication following strangles. Other infections and certain poisons can cause similar damage to the heart muscle. The sudden deaths that occasionally happen to racehorses at race meetings should also be mentioned in this connection. Post mortem examinations have in several cases shown that a horse has died as a result of paralysis of the heart muscle caused by a hidden infection. In the majority of such cases these were infections of the throat. Acute intestinal infections and gut twists can also lead to the rapid production of poisonous substances which damage the heart muscle. If the damage affects the sino-atrial node of the heart disturbances of the

ECG test

normal rhythm will occur. The heart may beat faster, some beats may be missed, and there may sometimes be extra beats.

If a horse is suffering from inflammation of the heart muscle it is important to allow it to rest for an adequate period while being given suitable treatment. Sometimes a month 'off work' may be enough, more often convalescence lasts for two or more months. Before the horse is put back in training the ECG should have returned to normal, and the ECG tests should be repeated at intervals. Sometimes inflammations of the heart can become chronic; the damage does not heal, and instead the inflamed tissue can become fibrous scar tissue.

Valvular heart disease. Other parts of the heart can also be damaged. In acute general infections the agent of infection can damage the inside of the heart muscle and the heart valves. The valves can become narrower so that the blood cannot pass through so easily, putting a strain on the heart. If the valves do not close properly the blood can to some extent flow backwards, which also causes more work for the heart muscle. The heart begins to enlarge and begins to use up its reserves of strength, which works fine as long as any reserves are left. Eventually the heart becomes so enlarged that its pumping ability is tangibly reduced. This is then a chronic heart condition which prevents the horse from being able to work again.

Rupture in the heart may affect either the auricles or the ventricles but is perhaps more common in the aorta close to the heart. It has been demonstrated that there is a weakness here in the wall of the aorta. When the blood pressure becomes abnormally high because of some considerable exertion the aorta ruptures and the horse dies in a matter of minutes from internal bleeding.

145

It may be of interest that the horse does not suffer from cholesterol deposition or arteriosclerosis of the heart.

Congenital heart disease does occur, but very rarely. The most usual deformity is in the walls between the various chambers of the heart. Often the foal is born weak and soon dies, though occasionally a foal with a minor heart deformity may survive.

MEDICAL INVESTIGATION OF TIREDNESS

Horses which become continually 'tired' should be very thoroughly examined. Apart from an ECG test they should be given a general medical examination, including listening to the heart and lungs, examination of the upper respiratory tract (nose, throat etc) by means of a special instrument, blood tests, and tests to determine the condition of the muscles, liver and nerves. The faeces should be examined for traces of parasite infestation. Usually the reason for the animal's lack of condition will be discovered and the correct treatment prescribed. The owner should follow carefully the vet's instruction regarding aftercare, and the horse should be re-examined before starting work again.

Many illnesses are often difficult for the horse-owner to detect in the early stages, but if one knows one's horse well and looks after it properly and regularly the chances of detecting the first symptoms of illness are far greater.

DISEASES OF THE GENITO-URINARY TRACT

KIDNEY DISEASES

The kidneys' functions include separating out water, salt and waste-products of the body's metabolism.

Inflammations in the kidneys are more common in omnivores than in herbivores, but purulent inflammations do occur as complications following suppuration elsewhere in the body, eg bastard strangles and purulent inflammations of the joints. Abscesses are often found in the kidneys of foals suffering from sleepy foal disease. Sometimes inflammations travel upwards from the bladder and the urethra. Other types of damage to the tissues of the kidneys may be caused by muscle inflammations, liver damage and poisoning. Sometimes old horses have chronic kidney disease, in which the kidneys increasingly lose their function, but general urea poisoning is rare.

Symptoms of kidney disease are increased thirst and loss of appetite. The volume of urine increases and the horse urinates frequently. Treatment with sulpha drugs and antibiotics can sometimes cure kidney infections.

Diabetes insipidus is a mysterious disease that manifests itself by an excessive thirst and the production of large amounts of urine, often affecting all the horses in a stable. It is possible that it is the result of poisoning caused by a mould. Sometimes it is treated with medicinal charcoal. The disease is normally cured by a change in the diet.

DISEASES OF THE URINARY TRACT

Inflammations of the urinary tract. *Inflammations of the bladder* (cystitis) are more usually seen in mares than in stallions. The symptoms are difficulty in passing urine and sometimes blood in the urine. If possible a bacterial culture test should be performed on a urine sample to determine a suitable sulpha drug or antibiotic treatment.

'Stones' in the bladder are encountered from time to time. The horse frequently takes up the urinating stance without producing more than a very small amount of urine. The 'stone' can be very large, in which case it must be removed by an abdominal operation.

Rupture of the bladder. During birth the foal's bladder – especially with male foals – may very occasionally be ruptured. Probably this happens when the foal's bladder is too full of urine and is pressed against the mare's pelvis during birth. The foal's owner may notice that the foal tries to urinate but only a few drops come out. The foal becomes

147

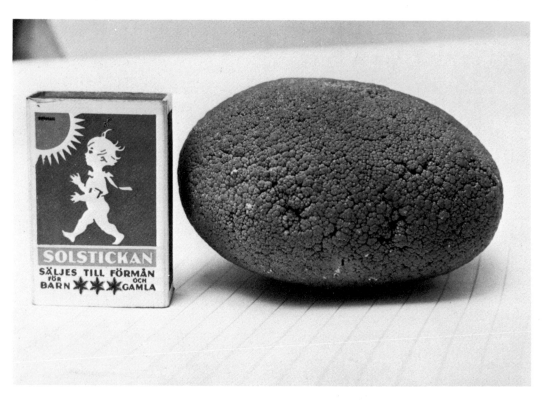

'Stone' taken from horse's bladder

uneasy and exhibits the symptoms of a mild colic, frequently lying down and getting up again. Slowly the abdomen fills with urine, becoming pear-shaped. If the foal is operated on as soon as possible the chances of recovery are good.

DISEASES OF THE GENITAL ORGANS

Tumours in the ovaries of mares often cause oestrus to be less marked or to be missed out altogether. The mare does not become pregnant. The tumour may reach a considerable size and can easily be felt by a *per rectum* examination. In the authors' experience only one ovary is affected, so that the outlook is good if the ovary is removed. The remaining ovary starts to function normally again, the mare comes on heat and as a rule becomes pregnant if she is covered.

A new highly infectious disease made its appearance in 1977 at many of the Thoroughbred studs in Newmarket, England. It was first seen in Ireland in 1976. The form of the disease is a highly contagious venereal disease of horses. The cause appears to be a bacterium hitherto not recognised, and causes violent inflammation of the genital organs of the mares. At the present time it is not clear how stallions are affected although they can carry it. Treatment is an intensive course of penicillin.

Tumours of the testicles are sometimes seen in old stallions. If the tumour only affects one side the operation to remove the tumour is likely to be successful, and there seems to be no tendency for the tumour to spread.

Injuries caused while the mare is being covered have become much more common recently. The causes vary, for example lack

148

of experience in handling stallions, a mare that shows very few signs when in heat, choosing too large a stallion for a small mare, etc.

Often such injuries occur when a mare is being covered for the first time. The damage is in the upper part of the vagina, where the mucous membrane can be split away over a varying area, causing copious bleeding. The mare strains and is in obvious discomfort. Small wounds can heal naturally but often surgery is necessary. It is not unknown for the larger arteries to be ruptured and the mare to die very quickly of internal bleeding. A complete rupture in the vulva can also cause peritonitis, also leading to the mare's death.

The penis can also be damaged, causing a permanent prolapse. The prognosis is poor.

COMPLICATED BIRTHS

Torsion or twisting of the uterus may occur during the later stages of pregnancy. The mare shows signs of having colic, but the symptoms are very moderate. Torsion can be diagnosed by *per rectum* examination. Operations to right the twist are usually successful; the mare does not abort, and the foal is born after the normal term without complications.

If torsion occurs when the birth is imminent a caesarean section may be necessary. Nowadays this operation need not cause a mare any great inconvenience. Other cases where a caesarean section are indicated include a serious mis-presentation, a deformed foetus or a dehydrated birth canal where the usual methods of assisting birth are not possible. Usually the foal's life cannot be saved, but the mare's chances of recovery are good, and she should also be able to conceive again.

Rupture of the rectum sometimes occurs during birth. During delivery the foal's fore-foot can easily go up into the top of the vagina and be pushed by the powerful contractions through the roof of the vagina into the rectum. This can cause either a recto-vaginal fistula or a vaginal prolapse. The damage may be extensive and a surgical repair should be done as soon as possible. Usually several operations are necessary before the cure is complete; the result is generally satisfactory. If the mare is attended while foaling the injury may possibly be prevented by correcting the position of the foal's fore-leg.

Mastitis occurs from time to time. It is important to examine the udder before the birth; if the foal drinks infected milk the consequences may be very serious. The mare's symptoms are obvious; the udder swells and the swelling often spreads forward under the abdomen. The udder becomes hard and the mare reacts with vigorous signs of discomfort when the udder is examined with the hand. The milk contains lumps and the mare has a raised temperature. Mastitis can occur before or at the time of birth, when the foal is being weaned and in mares that are not pregnant.

Treatment – bathing the udder, stripping the milk frequently and antibiotic treatment – must be started as soon as possible. In most cases the inflammation will be cured within a week. Widespread infections by *Botriomyces equi* may necessitate amputation of part of the udder.

Hyperlipemia, as the name suggests, is an abnormal build-up of fats (among others, cholesterol and triglycerides) in the blood. The condition occurs in mares either in the late stages of pregnancy or after foaling. The liver is severely damaged, and inadequate feeding is a contributory cause. In recent years we have observed this condition above all in horses in the categories mentioned above which have been exposed to some form of stress, such as long journeys and/or a change in environment and feeding. Most frequently affected are ponies that have been imported from Holland. The condition develops a day or so after arrival, and the first sign is a reduced appetite, soon followed by a complete lack of appetite. The horses develop fever and watery diarrhoea. In the opening stages of the condition the horses can drink, but quite soon they become unable to swallow. They show symptoms of severe thirst, standing with their muzzles submerged in the water bucket but unable to drink the water. They soon become lethargic and quite uninterested in their surroundings. In a newly taken blood sample a milk-white layer of fat can be observed at the top of the blood test tube a few minutes after the sample is taken.

The affected animals often die, but it is possible by an intensive and quite special type of treatment to save about 65 per cent of them.

Milk fever occurs especially in pony mares suckling foals 10–30 days after giving birth and when the horses are out on rich grazings in June. The disease is characterised by a stiff gait, a slightly raised tail, clenched jaws and trembling in the muscles of the shoulders and jaws. Rhythmic jerks run through the whole body in time with the heart-beats. The disease is reminiscent of lockjaw, and can be fatal unless speedily treated. Treatment is to administer a solution of calcium and magnesium salts directly into the bloodstream, and within ten minutes the mare is visibly better; within an hour she is usually completely back to normal.

CASTRATION

Castration is the removal of the testicles and associated structures. The aim of the operation is to create a more useful animal, as a gelding has a more amenable temperament than a stallion. Feeding, too, becomes simpler, for geldings can be allowed to graze with mares; this may be particularly important where there are several horses and a limited amount of land available for pasture.

It was formerly the custom to castrate working horses at around a year old, preferably in the spring, but recently there has been a tendency to wait until stallions are 3–4 years old. This is to allow them to develop a more massive, stallion-like build.

Trotters and Thoroughbreds are rarely castrated before they are 3–4 years old. This is partly because certain classic races are still not open to geldings, and also because stallions are supposed to be able to run better than geldings. (Although the legendary American trotter 'Greyhound' was a gelding, and he was the world record holder for several decades.)

Many stallions have very intractable temperaments, and they have to be castrated before they can become useful working animals. Sometimes horses have to be castrated for medical reasons, eg as a result of inflammations or tumours of the testicles, or scrotal hernia. It may sometimes be necessary to castrate a stallion with leg injuries that take a long time to heal, in order to make him calmer during convalescence.

Castrating a horse is usually a simple operation. It may be done to a standing horse under a local anaesthetic or to a horse lying down under a general anaesthetic. The authors are of the opinion that in cases where there is any risk of hernia a general anaesthetic is necessary. The operation is done under aseptic conditions, the spermatic cord is tied off and the incision sewn up. The risks of hernia are avoided, and the risk of infection minimised. As a rule the horse can be put back to work after a month.

In the writers' opinion many more stallions should be castrated than is at present the case, because so many horses are nowadays owned by youngsters with very little experience of horses.

SKIN DISEASES

IRRITATION

Lice. A horse that scratches itself should first of all be examined for lice. These appear in winter when the horse has long hair. Horses with lice often rub the hair from the region on either side of the tail and bite their flanks. Lice and eggs are usually found on the neck, under the mane, along the back and at the root of the tail.

De-lousing is done with a suitable preparation which is applied twice or three times at intervals of 10 days. All the horses in a stable must be de-loused at the same time as the stable is cleaned out and disinfected from top to bottom, not forgetting the grooming tackle. Young horses can be so seriously attacked by lice that they lose weight and become anaemic.

Foot mange or chorioptic mange occurs on the skin of the legs, mainly the hind-legs, and causes extreme irritation. Closer examination of the skin reveals a scurfy condition with loss of hair. The mites (*Chorioptes equi*) are easily seen under the microscope. Treatment is to wash the legs with a special shampoo that kills the mites. Stables, horse-brushes etc should also be disinfected.

True mange or sarcoptic mange causes loss of hair and great irritation over the whole body. This disease is now extinct in Sweden; the last occasion on which it was diagnosed was in 1940 on horses that had been imported from Hungary. When buying horses abroad one should always examine their skin. In the UK this is a notifiable disease, but it has not been seen for many years.

Ringworm or mycotic dermatitis is a fungal disease which causes a skin inflammation with round, hairless patches, and sometimes irritation.

The disease often takes an endemic form, ie is well distributed within a particular geographic area. It is mainly the younger animals which suffer from ringworm, and it can spread extremely fast, infecting a whole stable within a matter of days.

Horses with ringworm should not be brushed or combed but should just be dusted with clean dusters. The skin areas affected should be treated with appropriate medicaments. If the skin of the back or where the girths are fitted is affected, the horse should not be ridden until the skin has healed. Equine ringworm, like that of the other domesticated animals, can also affect humans, so it is sensible to take precautions when handling a horse with ringworm.

There are several other fungal infections of the horse's skin, such as Aspergillus, which can cause skin changes and irritation. The horse may bite its flanks, though the skin changes may seem insignificant. The veterinary surgeon will suggest treatment.

Sweet itch, a disease of which the cause is unknown, can cause extreme irritation in the mane and tail. It mostly affects ponies, often when put out to grass very early. The horses affected rub away the hair of the mane and tail, leaving the skin raw and scabby. Some horses seem predisposed to this disease, but the protein-rich spring grass and sunlight trigger it off. If the change to summer grazing is made as gradual as possible this helps. The ulcerated, scabby root of the tail and mane should be clipped free of hair and

Skin inflammation with widespread loss of hair caused by skin irritation

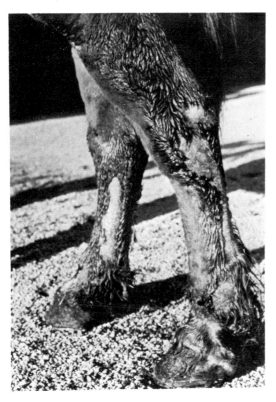

bathed, eg with an anti-dandruff shampoo, two or three times at weekly intervals. In some cases an anti-histamine preparation can help.

Irritation at the root of the tail may also be caused by Oxyuris (seatworms). When there is no apparent cause of the irritation bathing the area repeatedly with a soothing, antiseptic solution will remove the irritation.

Nettle-rash or urticaria appears as flat swellings on the skin of large areas of the body, usually accompanied by irritation. The cause can be unsuitable fodder or an allergy to a medicine, eg penicillin. The treatment is to remove the cause, give laxatives and an anti-histamine preparation.

SKIN TUMOURS

Warts. Tumours are not common in horses, but one does sometimes see small stalked warts on horses up to about three years old, most frequently on the muzzle or lips. These warts, which are caused by a virus, can number anything from one or two to several hundred. Usually they disappear spontaneously without treatment after a few months.

In some cases it may be necessary to remove the warts surgically. The virus which causes the warts enters the skin through small cuts; the warts appear 2–3 months after the infection. If they cause a lot of trouble in a stable year after year it is possible to produce a vaccine and vaccinate young animals that are not yet affected.

Sarcoids often begin as single hard lumps in the skin of the head, under the chest or abdomen, or on the udder or legs. The tumour breaks through the skin, developing an ulcerated surface, and gradually or sometimes rapidly grows, in some cases reaching a considerable size.

Horses may have only a single tumour, but they can have 20–30 varying from the size of a walnut to the size of two clenched fists. Although sarcoids do not spread to internal organs, they can be very difficult to treat.

The treatment is surgical. The risk of recurrence after the operation is high; the authors know of a case in which a horse needed seven operations before it was cured. The Animal Hospital in Helsingborg operates on about 30 horses with these tumours every year, and many of them need more than one operation. In rare cases the disease is incurable. It is believed that these tumours are caused by a virus; they can be produced experimentally by the transfer of a wart virus from a cow to damaged skin on a horse, and similarly warts can be produced in a cow by the transfer of material from a sarcoid on a horse. Sometimes the disease can be arrested by vaccination using a vaccine prepared from sarcoid tumour material, and we always vaccinate after surgery now. Sometimes horses with recurrent sarcoids recover spontaneously when taken to another part of the country.

Ringworm on flank and thigh

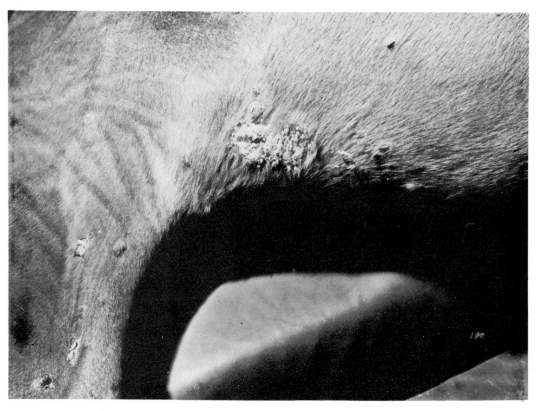

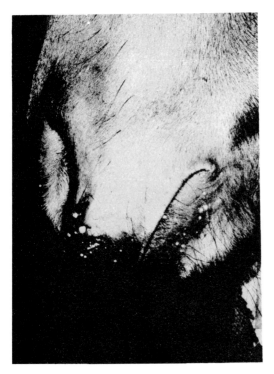

Warts

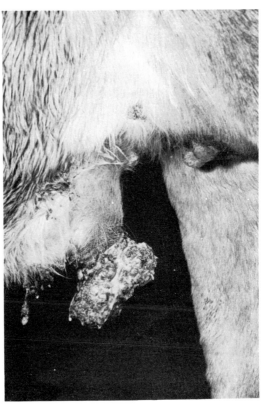

Sarcoid tumour

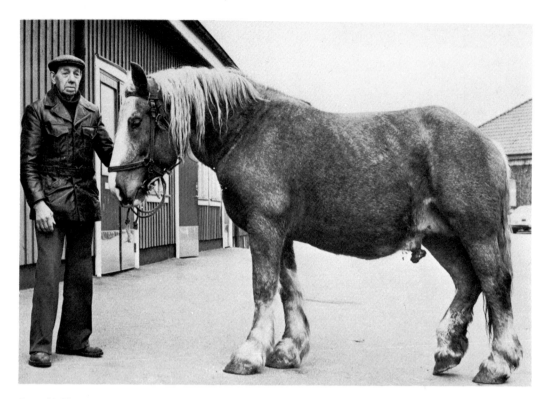

Sarcoid Tumour

EYE DISEASES

The normal eye. The function of the eye is to convey light impulses from the external world to the horse.

The transparent cornea, lens, aqueous humour and vitreous humour break up the light into an image on the retina. The eye can adjust its capacity to break up light according to its requirements. In the retina the light is changed photo-chemically into nerve impulses that the optic nerve then carries to optical centres in the back part of the brain, where the image is registered. Naturally enough a great deal about the horse's powers of sight can never be known to us. The horse's retina does not follow a regular curve, and the shape of the lens cannot be altered to focus the image. The focus is obtained by head and eye movements. We do not know whether horses have colour vision, though a horse can, for example, react to different colours on jumps. A blue jump is a more serious obstacle to a horse than a red one.

Eye deformities. Sometimes foals are born with deformed eyes. Instead of the normal eyeball there may be a very small eyeball or none at all, just small slits where the eye should be.

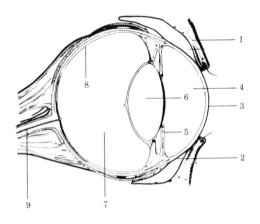

The horse's eye 1 Eyelid 2 Sclerotic coat 3 Cornea 4 Front chamber with aqueous humour 5 Iris 6 Lens 7 Vitreous humour 8 Retina 9 Optic nerve

Entropion is an inward folding of the eyelid. It can be congenital or a complication following other eye diseases. The hair-covered outside of the eyelid comes into contact with the cornea and can damage it. The horse has an excessive flow of tears and becomes photophobic. Soon the cornea develops a greyish discolouration. At first the damage is external but it gradually becomes deeper and more serious. Plastic surgery corrects the eyelid's tendency to roll in, and the damaged cornea soon heals.

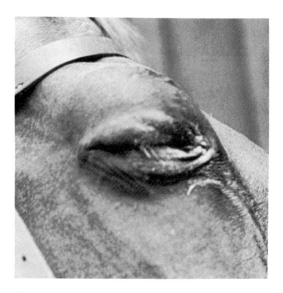
Entropion (inversion of eyelid)

Accidental eye damage such as lacerated wounds is most common on the upper eyelid. If the accident happens while the horse is out to grass it may be some time before it is noticed, which may make treatment more difficult. For best results cut eyelids should always be sutured; otherwise deformed or improperly closing eyelids can cause further damage to the eye. If the stitches burst a second plastic operation should be carried out to correct the defect.

Tumours on the eyelids are not uncommon. They are mainly warts which occur on the upper eyelid. During their surgical removal it is sometimes necessary to remove so much skin that plastic surgery is needed to achieve a satisfactory cosmetic result.

Cancer of the third eyelid can be very treacherous because at first it looks like a cut. It can grow rapidly and spread to the entire eye. In the early stages the diseased third eyelid is removed; in more advanced cases the whole eye must be extirpated. There is a risk of recurrence.

Deformed tear ducts. The eye is protected and kept moist by the tears which are secreted by the lacrimal glands which are above and to the outside of the eyes. Blinking conveys the tears across the eyeball and they collect in the lacrimal sac in the inside corner of the eye and are drained away by the tear ducts which open into the nostrils. Deformities can occur in which the opening to the nostrils is missing, or even part of the tear duct, in which case the tears are seen to run down the outside of the cheek.

Inflammation in the tear duct often occurs in connection with inflammation of the conjunctiva. The tear ducts are examined and treated by syringing from the nose.

Foreign bodies in the eye. The horse's owner may notice that it screws up its eyes. The flow of tears increases, the horse becomes photophobic and obviously uncomfortable. Objects that can get into the eye include chaff, straw, soil etc. We have even come across a horse that had been shot at with a shot-gun with a pellet in its eye.

To prevent damage to the cornea it is necessary to get help quickly. The first place to look for an object is under the third eyelid.

Inflammation of the conjunctiva is common in horses. On hot summer days the horse is pestered by flies which alight in the corners of the eyes. They often cause a pronounced inflammation (conjunctivitis) with reddening and swelling; inflammation can also be caused by bacteria, viruses, foreign bodies and poisonous substances.

Symptoms. The horse is photophobic (light-shy) and screws its eye up. The conjunctiva is red and swollen. The blood vessels are enlarged. The tears are clear at first but later mixed with pus.

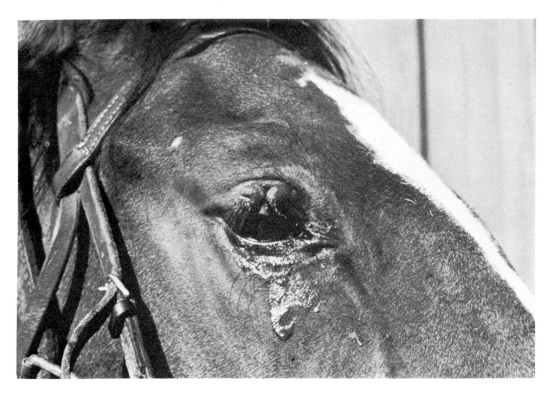

Cut eyelid

Inflammation of the cornea (keratitis) caused by parasites

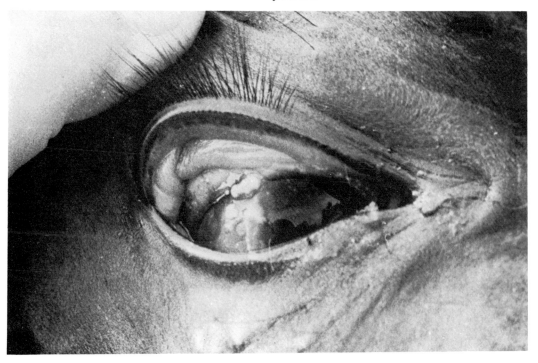

Treatment. Normally the conjunctiva with the help of the tears can resist less serious inflammations. The eye should be bathed with a weak solution of boracic acid at body temperature several times a day. If the inflammation is purulent sulpha drugs or antibiotics in the form of ointment or drops should be applied to the eye. The treatment should be repeated at least 5–6 times a day as the tears wash away the medicaments.

Inflammation of the cornea. When the inflammation spreads to the cornea the horse suffers even more discomfort. The eye is kept closed. Often the cornea becomes cloudy and whiteish-grey in colour. At a more advanced stage the blood-vessels of the conjunctiva spread into the cornea, which otherwise lacks blood-vessels. This corneal inflammation is very serious because the clouding of the cornea causes deterioration of the eyesight. The treatment, too, can often be very prolonged. Flies can cause widespread damage to the cornea, larvae hatching on the eye causing deep ulcers in the cornea. The inflammation takes a long time to heal and can last for several months; it can also easily lead to a general eye inflammation. For this reason atropine drops should always be used in the treatment of corneal inflammations and cuts to the cornea.

Wounds on the cornea. Wounds on the cornea can also cause it to cloud over. The extent of the wound is examined with the help of a pigment, fluorescein, which sticks to the damaged tissue. If the horse is photophobic it should be kept in a dark stable. Prolonged medical treatment is necessary. Extensive cuts should be sutured where possible; early surgery can give good results, even if a scar remains. If the damage is extensive and suturing therefore impossible, the third eyelid is drawn over the eye and sutured, thus effec-

tively protecting the wound. After 7–10 days the third eyelid is released. If the damage to the cornea is deep and extensive an inflammation of the whole eye can easily develop, and in some cases there may be no alternative but to remove the eye surgically. Glass eyes can be made and fitted, but this is rarely done. A one-eyed horse does not seem to be particularly handicapped; there are many cases of such horses being successful as trotters and show jumpers.

Cataract. Horses sometimes have congenital cataract, which makes the eye lens opaque. Cataract can be present at birth or develop during the first year of life. It can be inherited, and often other changes in the eye tissue take place at the same time, particularly in the iris. Cataract can also be caused by trauma or by eye inflammations.

Congenital cataract often takes the form of small areas of opacity in the lens, often only affecting one eye. Often the condition remains stable, in other cases it may progress until the affected eye becomes completely blind.

Cataract caused by trauma is not usually progressive. Medical treatment does not help; there is a surgical operation which is not often performed, and should only be recommended if the horse is blind.

Moon blindness has been recognised since the sixth century. The disease is characterised by inflammations of the parts of the eye that are richest in blood vessels, ie the vascular coat, the iris and the ciliary body. Moon blindness recurs at intervals, the horse's sight deteriorating after each attack. Typical symptoms are that the horse becomes markedly photophobic, the lens becomes opaque, pus collects in the front chamber and the cornea becomes opaque. In time the horse becomes blind. The disease is incurable, but its progression may be slowed by medical treatment.

This disease can have a variety of causes.

Eye examinations should be an important part of any medical examination. The eye is easily accessible, and eye examinations, apart from revealing eye diseases, can often reveal other general diseases. Lockjaw, for example, causes spasm of the third eyelid; anaemia causes the mucous membranes of the eye to become pale, and jaundice turns them yellow.

MALFORMATIONS

Malformations affecting horses' heads are mainly either of the teeth or jaws.

Undershot jaw (parrot mouth) results in the front teeth of the upper jaw being further forward than the front teeth of the lower jaw. In very serious cases the horse may have difficulty grazing. This malformation should be taken extremely seriously when judging horses that are intended for breeding purposes. A horse with undershot jaw will need regular dental checks for its whole life; the hooks that develop on the cheek teeth will need to be filed off once or twice a year.

Overshot jaw is also hereditary but less common. Foals with overshot jaws may have difficulty suckling. The same strictures apply as for undershot jaw.

Sometimes a foal is born with a congenital deformity of the front part of the upper jaw so that the front teeth in the upper and lower jaws lie side by side instead of meeting. Such animals should obviously not be used for breeding purposes. It may be worth attempting to correct the upper jaw by means of an operation.

Malformations of the mouth often prevent the teeth from meeting properly, leading to uneven wear and the impaction of food residues between the teeth, followed by tooth decay and inflammations in the root cavities.

Cleft palate is occasionally seen in foals. The deformity can affect the roof of the mouth, the soft palate or both. The foal always has difficulty in suckling. The milk runs out through the nostrils and the foal loses weight. Surgery may be attempted, but the operation is complicated and must be done in stages. The chances of a completely successful repair are not good.

Congenital ear fistula is a malformation typical of the horse. The cause is a deformed tooth that has developed in the wrong place in the foetus, usually on the frontal bone just below the base of the ear. The fistula runs from the tooth to an opening at the base of the ear or at the inner edge of the external ear. The owner may notice that the hair is matted because of the discharge from the fistula and that flies collect there in the summer. The malformation can be corrected satisfactorily by surgery.

Deformities of the gut are sometimes found in foals. Usually the large intestine or the

162

rectum are affected. The foal will have colic from birth because the meconium will be obstructed. Minor deformities can be corrected surgically.

Scrotal and umbilical hernia are often inherited defects present when foals are born. In the case of scrotal hernia the foal has too wide an opening in the groin so that the intestines can find their way down into the scrotum. Umbilical hernia is similar. Usually surgical treatment is necessary. Scrotal hernia is commonest in American trotters.

Rig or cryptorchid is a state in which one or both testicles have remained in the abdomen. Normally both testicles are in the scrotum at birth or descend shortly afterwards. They may also remain in the canal between the abdomen and the scrotum. The condition is commonest in ponies but does occur in various breeds of horse and is a very serious fault when a horse is judged. The testicles of stallions that are to be used for breeding must be very carefully examined; since the defect is hereditary such stallions are not suitable for stud purposes.

Treatment. A rig is often a very intractable animal, and should be castrated. Both descended and undescended testicles should be removed.

Extra feet. Occasionally a horse is born with an extra (supernumerary) foot. It is always on the inside of either a fore- or hind-leg. Sometimes it may be a horn-covered structure the size of a thumb, sometimes a fully developed foot with tendons, blood-vessels and nerves. The foot should be removed when the foal is at least a month old; the result is usually satisfactory.

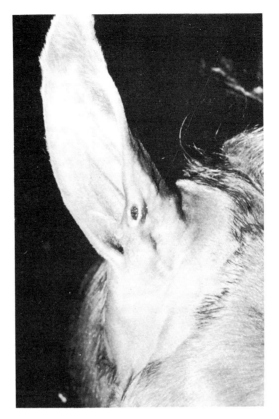

Congenital ear fistula

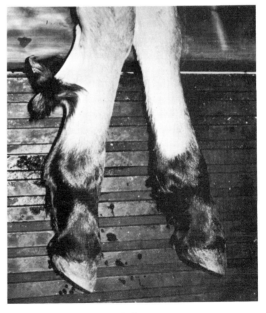

Extra (supernumerary) foot

163

VICES

A vice is a departure from normal behaviour that can damage either the horse or its surroundings.

Vices may appear at almost any period of a horse's life. Thus crib-biting may begin before a foal is weaned. Vices may be caused by nervousness, neglect, being ill at ease, overtrained, or not being given enough to do. Vices may occur spontaneously, or be learnt from other horses. Heredity may also predispose to certain vices. To control a vice one must first try to remove the possible causes at the earliest stages – regular exercise, being well looked after and getting plenty of time outdoors are important. Start to handle and to bring up the horse while it is still a foal.

Crib-biting is a vice in which the horse grasps the edge of the manger or other object with with its front teeth and then swallows air, making a gulping sound. There are various opinions about the causes of crib-biting; some say it gives the horse a pleasurable sensation, others that it is a neurosis comparable with aerophagia (swallowing air) in humans. Some horses develop the vice when foals, others may learn it from a crib-biting horse that comes to the stable.

Some horses suffer no ill-effects from this vice, but most suffer digestive disorders, and lose weight and condition. The constant gulping noise is very irritating to the animal's owner. Crib-biting is commonest in Thoroughbreds and in saddle horses. It is sometimes seen in ponies but very rarely in Trotters. As already mentioned, there may be an hereditary predisposition. One investigation showed, among other things, that a certain Thoroughbred stallion had many crib-biters among his progeny.

Treatment. Many traditional remedies exist, such as the cribbing strap, but none of them are particularly reliable. The best method is an operation introduced by Professor Gerhard Forssell more than fifty years ago. Briefly, the operation is to remove parts of the muscles which control the movements of the throat when swallowing air. The operation is usually successful; a follow-up of 130 horses operated on by the Animal Hospital in Helsingborg, Sweden, showed that the operation had cured the horses of this vice in 90 per cent of the cases. Horses most likely to relapse, according to the survey, were those that had been crib-biters for a long time.

The horse's owner is therefore advised to

164

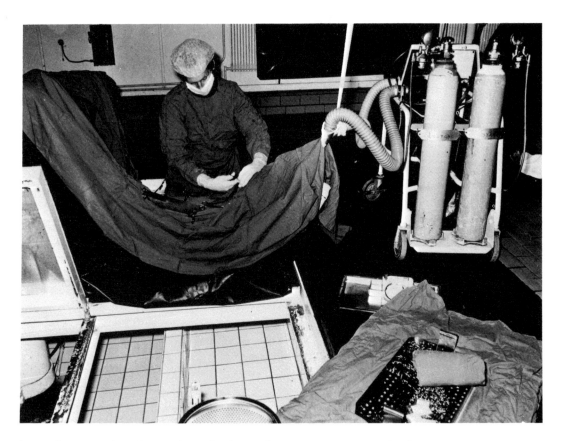

Operating on a crib-biter

have the operation done when the horse is about three years old. The operation saves the horse much discomfort and prevents other horses from learning this vice.

Until the horse is old enough to have the Forssell operation carried out it should be discouraged from practising its vice by means of suitable fences, stable fittings, and possibly by trying the cribbing strap.

Windsucking is another form of aerophagia in horses. This vice is very similar to crib-biting except that the horse does not support itself with its teeth. It is a fairly unusual vice. Here, too, a Swedish method of treatment has been introduced. Professor Gunnar Tufvesson, of the Swedish Veterinary Institute, and the veterinarian Sigvard Karlander of Karlstad, have shown that the vice can be cured surgically. This method prevents the horse from creating a vacuum in the mouth by the insertion of metal canulae in the cheeks. The horse can then no longer swallow air.

Chewing wood. Horses quite often chew fences or stable fittings. The cause may be tooth trouble, stomach or intestinal parasites or mineral deficiency, but probably the most common causes are boredom, nervousness or too little exercise. First of all one should try to remove possible causes, before trying putting a wire along the top rail of the fences, perhaps slightly electrified, and plating vulnerable parts of the stable with sheet metal. If pine logs are put in the paddock with their branches and leaves still on, the horses eat these instead of chewing wood.

165

Weaving is seen particularly in highly strung Thoroughbreds in very good condition stabled at racetracks. Weaving may arise spontaneously or be learnt from other horses.

The horse shifts from side to side on its fore-legs for shorter or longer periods, during which the fore-quarters swing like a pendulum. This puts an unnatural strain on the fore-legs and can damage joints and tendons. In general the horse tends to lose its appetite, lose weight and go out of condition.

Treatment aims to make the horse calmer by improving conditions in the stable and regular exercise. Sedatives can also be given when the horse is resting.

Circling is a similar vice. The horse continually walks round in a circle in the loose-box. The same kind of damage may be done as with weaving, and roughly the same treatment is recommended. Tying the horse may also help.

Vices of temperament. Some horses kick and bite. Everyone who has anything to do with such horses must be told about their temperaments, so that they can be ready to defend themselves in case of a sudden attack.

All too often one comes across horses that have not been properly treated and looked after while they were growing up. Such horses can be difficult to break in and also very difficult for the vet to examine and treat. Often these horses kick viciously; they may kick forwards, cow fashion, with the hind-legs. One should always be careful when handling a horse with which one is **not** familiar.

BUYING AND IMPORTING

Buying the right horse is a difficult art. There are few people fortunate enough to have the intuitive gift that enables them time after time to obtain horses that develop into first-class show-jumping or dressage horses, trotters or racehorses. Most buyers, and in particular all novices, should seek the help of an expert on the type of horse they wish to buy.

A veterinary examination should also be made when buying a horse, preferably by the vet who will later have the job of looking after the horse. This is a custom which ought to be made into a rule. There are many reasons for this. The buyer's vet knows his client and his standard of horsemanship, and at the same time future conflicts and discussions are avoided. Remember that there are no strict biological frontiers between the normal and the abnormal, and different vets will not attach the same amount of importance to any abnormalities they notice. If the vet has recommended buying the horse, it will be in his interest to cure the horse if afterwards it shows symptoms of disease.

When buying a horse disregard any old veterinary certificates. A horse, like any other living creature, can injure itself or become ill immediately after a veterinary examination.

Many prospective buyers of horses think that taking a vet along as an adviser when buying a horse should be sufficient, but it should be remembered that being a skilled veterinarian and a good judge of horseflesh is an unusual combination.

Often the seller may ask a high price so that there is plenty of room for bargaining, thereby letting the buyer delude himself into thinking that he has made a very good bargain by getting so much knocked off the asking price.

As soon as the horse is bought it should be insured. It is also important that the horse is given sufficient time to get accustomed to its new surroundings, its new fodder, new work, etc. One should take care to find out how the horse was stabled, that there were no infectious diseases present there, how it was fed and worked, etc.

Buying a horse in a foreign country demands considerable ability in the buyer or access to a very expert adviser. To import a horse to the UK a special permit is required, issued by the Ministry of Agriculture, who will in each individual case lay down certain conditions to be complied with according to the diseases that may be endemic in the horse's country of origin.

ACKNOWLEDGEMENTS

The publishers would like to thank Mr P. J. Waters MRCVS and Miss Daphne Machin Goodall for their kindness in checking the translation of the text.

Black and white photographs: Pelle Norén, Västerås, p11; Arne Eilert, Kolbäck, pp12, 41, 44; Lasse Rudberg, Västerås, pp17, 18, 19, 20, 21, 22; Flash-Photo, Malmö, pp30, 31, 32, 35; Christer Linnaeus, Västerås, p63; Bertil Persson, Lindbergs Foto Eftr, Helsingborg, pp48, 49, 50, 51, 52, 53, 54, 55, 71, 74, 75, 79, 80, 81, 82, 83, 84, 87, 88, 89, 92, 93, 95, 99, 119, 123, 124, 125, 126, 127, 132, 138, 142, 145, 154, 156, 160, 165; Anita Franzeén, Växjö, p155; all other black and white photographs by courtesy of the Animal Hospital, Helsingborg.

Colour photographs: parasites series by AB Teknosan, Malmö; birth series by Wåge Palerby, Kolbäck; all other colour photographs by courtesy of the Animal Hospital, Helsingborg.

The photograph on the front of the jacket was taken by Sven Jönsson, Stockholm.

Line drawings by Christina Kämärä, Västerås, after (pp6 and 9) Helmut Ende, *Die Stallapotheke,* Ruschlikon-Zurich 1971; (p7) *Instruktion för arméns hovslagarmanskap,* Stockholm 1949; (p8) Ellenberger and Baum, *Handbuch der vergelichden Anatomie der Haustiere,* Berlin 1926.

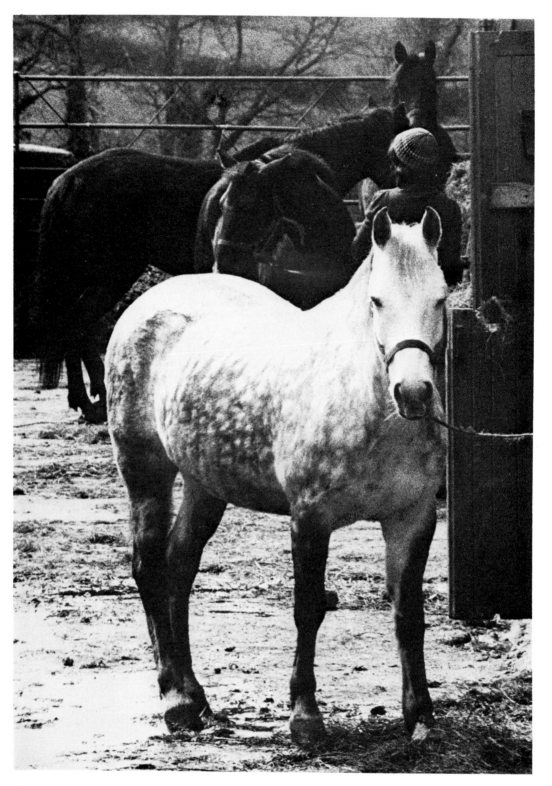

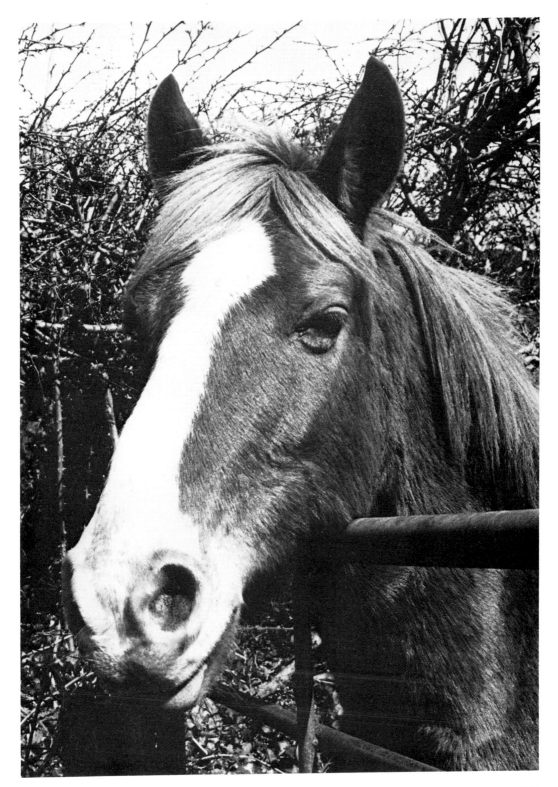

INDEX

Page numbers in italic type indicate illustrations.

176